CHINESE MEDICINE 102: COMPLETE YOUR FOUNDATIONS

Part two of a two-part journey into understanding Chinese Medicine

By Cat Calhoun, MAcOm, L.Ac.

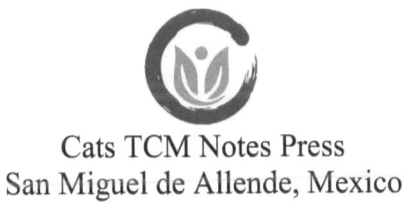

Cats TCM Notes Press
San Miguel de Allende, Mexico

This page intentionally left blank

For DeLora, my sunshine and my rest
Thank you with all my heart for your supporting
and for sticking with me through Chinese Medicine School!

This page intentionally left blank

Table of Contents

Chinese Medicine 102: Complete your Foundations

ACKNOWLEDGMENTS

No one does anything truly on their own. I thought myself totally self-sufficient before I dove into the study of Chinese medicine. When that journey began, my eyes opened to the myriads of those who were actively helping me, those who have gone before, and even those who will come long after I'm gone. We are interconnected. You are me, I am you.

I especially want to thank Dr. Qianzhi Wu, my teacher and one of the wisest souls I have ever encountered. Thank you for your wisdom and your teaching, for your patience and guidance, for the gift of Qigong which I would not have seen with the beauty that it is without you showing it to me.

Thank you to Master Junfeng Li, my Shengzhen Qigong teacher. Qigong kept me sane and healthy in school and for this I thank you.

Thank you to Lisa Lapwing, a most awesome practitioner based in Orlando Florida. We studied together, practiced together, we practiced *on* each other in student clinic, and then we became each others' practitioners! Not having Lisa in my daily life is my one giant regret about moving to Mexico.

Thank you to my buds: Donna "Needles" Tatum, Tiffany Chiu Peralez, Vanessa Olsen, Andi Kohn, Mark Hernandez, and Katherine Webster. To Georgie Hoiseth, a kick ass practitioner and fellow computer geek, I thank thee! To Rita Ramirez, I would *NOT* want to be on this journey without you!

And to so may more who have loved, supported, and believed in me, I express my gratitude and thanks. May the deity of your choice look favorably upon you all!

Cat Calhoun

This page intentionally left blank

SECTION 1: VITAL SUBSTANCES

There are two categories of body things in Chinese medicine for which you won't find many equivalents in biomedicine: Vital Substances and the Three Treasures.

Vital Substances are actually visible things, while the Three Treasures are not visible to the eye. Vital substances include Essence, Qi, Blood, and Body Fluids. The Three Treasures are Essence, Qi, and Shen. And yes, Qi makes a strong showing in both categories.

I should point out that the Maciocia books says Shen is a Vital Substance, but all of my professors disagreed. In China Vital Substances are all visible and observable. Shen, a mental activity, is not directly viewable.

Why am I listening to my professors instead of Maciocia? They've all studied Chinese medicine in China in Chinese for minimum of 30 years each and collectively have logged an impressive 2+ centuries of study and publication on this stuff. I'm going with the profs!

This page intentionally left blank

CHAPTER 1:

Essence

In Chinese medicine, Essence is called "Jin" and is written as a combination of the glyphs for "rice" and "green." Essence is a fluid-like vital substance, the most basic and important of the vital substances to the body. Transformation of all other vital substances relies on essence.

> *Essence is a fluid-like substance, the most basic and important of the vital substances to the body.*

By broad definition, Essence is a compilation of *all* vital substances in the human body, including the narrow definition of Blood and Qi and Body Fluids. By narrow definition, Essence is a fluid-like vital substances such as sperm or an egg. For the purposes of this discussion, we will use the narrow definition.

TYPES OF ESSENCE

There are two types of Essence to know.
- Congenital, Prenatal, or Pre-Heaven Essence
  This is your starter pack, courtesy of your parents. You only get a specific amount so don't spend it all in once place!

- Acquired, Postnatal, or Post-Heaven Essence
  This is what you acquire from your food, water, air, and Qi or prana-building exercises (such as yoga and qigong).

Both types of Essence are *stored* in the Kidneys, even though the Spleen is the *root* (or source) of Post-Heaven Essence. Acquired Essence supports and tonifies the congenital Essence. Even if you have good congenital Essence you can "overspend" it by over working and be worn out in mid to late life.

If you build good acquired Essence, you will not have to dip so deeply into the pool of congenital Essence.

FUNCTIONS OF ESSENCE

If you remember the discussion on the Kidney from *Chinese Medicine 101: Start with the Foundations*, Chapter 9 (available on Amazon in both digital and print formats), you will remember that we talked quite a bit about Essence. That's because the Kidney and Essence are so tied together.

Essence is like a building block that can be converted into Qi or into Yin. Essence converts to primary or Yuan Qi and then to Kidney qi. Essence can also be transformed into Kidney yin while the Kidney Qi can transform into Kidney yang. Primary Qi (or Yuan Qi) can be transformed into any kind of organ Qi, working on the organ which then produces that type of Qi.

Know this diagram and/or this concept!

Essence	☞	Yuan Qi	☞	Kidney Qi
👇				👇
Kidney Yin		☞ ☞		Kidney Yang

These are the functions of essence:

Growth, reproduction, and development

We spoke about this at length during the discussion on the Kidney and Urinary Bladder in the previous book. Please see that text for more detailed information. (*Chinese Medicine 101: Start with the Foundations*, available on Amazon in both digital and print formats.)

Essence is the basis of Kidney qi, as reflected in the diagram.

Essence converts into Yuan Qi and then is differentiated into Kidney Qi

Essence produces Marrow (brain, bone, and spine)

The brain is the Sea of Marrow. Good essence → good marrow → strong bones → good brain function. Alzheimer's, senility, and dementia are all examples of depletion of the Kidney essence. Eat your bone soup. Bone soup nourishes both marrow and essence. See the recipe in the previous book! (*Chinese Medicine 101: Start with the Foundations*, available on Amazon in both digital and print formats.) It's so much better than anything I've bought off of the shelf!

Actually, the Chinese traditional way is to eat whatever it is that's weak: weak Kidneys? Eat some kidneys. Bad eyes? Eat some liver since Liver controls the eyes. This is no longer recommended because of antibiotics and the generally toxic environment in which most food animals live. (And also because liver is gross, but that's just my opinion.)

To tonify Qi and Blood, animal herbs are, as a rule, more effective than plants…bummer for your vegetarian patients. Some herbal professors will tell you to just keep it a secret from them and add the ingredients into the formula anyway, but I disagree. They need to be informed and they need to know that the vegetarian option will work more slowly. Let them decide, don't do it for them.

Essence is the basis of constitutional strength.

Again, this is tied to Kidneys. If the constitution is poor at birth, it's a good bet the Essence is too.

This page intentionally left blank.

CHAPTER 2:
Qi

The Chinese character for Qi is the character for vapor over the character for rice. Rice and vapor represents the process of cooking.

Qi can be **seen** – in food via the vapor of cooking, in the human body through the vapor formed by the breath when it is cold. Cloud forests will also show you their Qi in the vapor and mist. We've probably all seen vapor rising up on a cold morning, or in a tropical forest. . . or even when you breathe out on a cold morning and see the fog created by your exhale. You can **smell** Qi. Good food smells, bad food smells, body odors, etc. are all the smell of Qi. This the active essence, reaching out to 'touch' your nasal sensors whether you want them to or not!

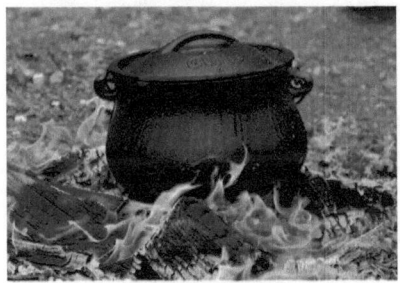

Essence produces Qi. At the beginning of the Essence chat above, I mentioned that it is fluid-like. The heat of the Mingmen "vaporizes" this fluid-like Essence and converts it into Qi. In the photograph, the pot represents our store of Essence. The fire is the Mingmen fire which is said to reside between the Kidneys is represented by . . . well, by the fire!

When the fire of the Mingmen heats the stored Essence, it produces Yuan Qi, a type of Qi building block, which can then be refined and molded into the specific Qi that is associated with the organs. The oxygen fueling the combustion energy of the fire is the Lungs and the breath.

Fun thing to know: Qigong can help you build Qi. Check out the Six Healing Sounds Qigong to strengthen the Qi of the various Yin organs in the body. Qigong requires regulation of the mind (fire), regulation of the breath (oxygen) and regulation of the physical body – represented by the oven and the pot and its contents.

There are several levels of Qigong:
- ☯ Transportation of the Essence into Qi
- ☯ Transportation of the Qi to the Shen
- ☯ Transportation of the Shen to the Universe.

That is the goal of Qigong: to re-combine yourself with the universe.

KNOW THIS ABOUT QI!

1. Qi can be seen, smelled, and strengthened through Qigong.

2. Definition of Qi:
   - Qi is a refined energy, produced by the internal organs, which has the function of nourishing the physical body and the mind. It is part of the vital substances.
   - Qi indicates the functional activities of the internal organs. All internal organ Qi derives from the essence of the Kidneys.

3. Source of Qi:
   - Da Qi - Air - Da, Dan or Big Qi.
     It is also called Qing Qi, Dan Qi and Big Qi.
     Da Qi comes from the Heavens and is related to the Lungs.

   - Gu Qi
     Food or Gu Qi is a collective term. It is made up of Ying/Nutritive Qi and Wei/Protective/Defensive Qi.
     It is from the Earth and is related to the Spleen.

   - Yuan Qi
     This is the Congenital or Primary Qi and comes from your parents. This is a fixed and limited

amount and is the most important dose of Qi you have.

> Side note: you can also get Qi from nature – you learn that in Qigong classes in which you do a meditation and visualize Qi entering your pores, clinging to your hands, entering your Dantian, etc. You must open up your channels in order to get Qi from nature. Please note that you can also get unhealthy Qi from your clients unless you learn to shield yourself from it. Qigong can help with this too.

DIFFERENCES BETWEEN ESSENCE AND QI

Essence	Qi
Fluid like	Energy like
Stored in the Kidneys	Runs everywhere
Located deep in the body	Is more superficial
Static – because it must be stored	Dynamic – because it must go everywhere
Hard to replenish/strengthened Essence, Blood and Yin are all difficult to replenish. Can take up to a year to replenish Yin with food, herbs, acutherapy	Easily tonified Qi and Yang bounce back quickly. Beware of too much Qi, causing hyperfunction and fire
Essence is Yin in nature	Qi is Yang in nature.

Staying up late consistently, addictions, and overeating *deplete* the Essence.

DIFFERENT TYPES OF QI

The Neijing says there are *eighty three* types of Qi! Eighty three!! You aren't expected to memorize that many, but there are a few types you do need to know:

Primary or Yuan Qi

Primary or Yuan Qi derives from Kidney Essence. Primary Qi is stored/located in the Mingmen, which is the space between the two Kidneys. In older written sources – before the 13th century – the right Kidney was thought to be the dwelling place of Primary Qi. Other sources say it is located in the Dantian (red elixir field) in the lower abdomen and this is correct as well.

Yuan Qi has several functions:
- It is the motivating force, supporting the activities of the whole body and supporting life.

- It is the basis of Kidney Qi

- It facilitates the transformation of Qi

- It facilitates the transformation of Blood
  Spleen and Stomach produce and move the body fluids to the Lungs which sends them to the Heart to make red Blood. The Yuan Qi provides the Heart with the energy to create Heart Qi which makes and drives the Blood. It is the Kidney Essence which supplies the material components needed to create Blood. So as you can see, you gotta have healthy Kidneys and Spleen to have a healthy Heart and Blood.

- Yuan Qi comes out at the Yuan Source Points
  Each channel/meridian has a yuan primary point or source point. You use these points to tonify the organs. The back shu points are used in combination with them in order to powerfully tonify the organs as well.

Some ways to tonify the Yuan Qi:
- Acupuncture
  o Tonify the primary source points on the channel
  o Tonify Ren 4 and Ren 6 at the Lower Dantian
  o Tonify Du 4 on the spine at L2 to tonify both Kidneys and Mingmen
- Diet and Herbs
  Foods like bone soup and herbs such as ren shen
- Qigong!

Gu Qi, aka Food Qi

There are two types of Gu Qi: Wei (protective) Qi and Ying (nutritive) Qi. Note that Maciocia says there is only one kind. My Chinese professors disagree. Guess who I'm inclined to listen to! Yeah, the Chinese people who studied Chinese medicine in China in Chinese for 20 years.

Gu Qi is derived from the Spleen and Stomach, the earth element. To get more specific, Ying Qi comes from the Spleen. Wei Qi, the defensive Qi, comes from the Stomach. Why? Because nutritive Qi (Ying) is very Yin oriented and is thus associated with the Yin organ. Wei Qi is more Yang in nature and is therefore associated with the Stomach organ.

Ying or Nutritive Qi

If you could literally find Ying Qi, you would see it hanging out inside the Blood vessels. Ying Qi is one of two ingredients in Blood; the other is Body Fluids. Blood is produced in the Heart from materials supplied by the Spleen. Though Ying and Body Fluids are both colorless, the red color of Blood is said to come from the elemental color of the Heart: red.

There are two main functions of Ying Qi:
- Nourish the internal organs and body tissues
- Moisten the soft tissues and the internal organs.

Defending or Wei Qi

Wei Qi is located between the soft tissues of the skin and muscle, but outside of the Blood vessels. It is considered more superficial (and therefore more Yang in nature) than Ying Qi because of its' location.

The three main functions of Wei Qi are:
1. Nourish and moisten the soft tissues of the skin and muscles

2. Defend the body by preventing invasion by external pathogens
3. Control the opening and closing of the sweating pores to maintain body temperature

Note: when one has a cold, the Wei Qi is blocked, causing have fever and chills. Promote sweating to move the Wei Qi where it needs to be, to regulate body temperature and to sweat out toxins.

Differences between Wei Qi and Ying Qi

Both are related to the bioclock and both are carriers of the Mind and Shen.

Ying Qi	Wei Qi
Sticky, turbid part of the food essence	Clear, light part of the food essence
Static, flows slowly with the Blood	Dynamic
Flows in the Blood vessels, is more localized and deeper	Flows outside of the Blood vessels, more generalized, more superficial, runs everywhere.
Yin in nature	Yang in nature

Both are related to the bioclock and both are carriers of the Mind and Shen.

In many acupuncture systems, there are three depth layers for acupuncture points. Different types of Qi are said to flow at each layer.
1. First layer = **Wei Qi** flow
   When the Wei Qi layer is stimulated, the skin reddens and/or twitches.
   If your patient has an infectious illness, do not penetrate below the wei Qi layer or you could push the disease into the body further.

2. Second layer = **Ying Qi** flow
   A heavy or deep sensation indicates the tapping

and manipulation of Ying Qi.

3. Third layer = **Yuan Qi** flow
   A suction or holding sensation indicates you
   have stimulated the Yuan or Primary Qi.

The sensations at the site of needle insertion are connected with Qi flow and thus metal needles conduct the flow best.

Skin that "tents" up around the needle can indicate an excess. If the skin depresses at the insertion site around the needle it can indicate a deficiency.

If you get a needle stuck in the skin and it won't let go, put another needle into the skin close to it so that the Wei Qi flows to it and spreads out the energy. Then remove both needles.

Zong Qi

Zong Qi is also called Gathering Qi or Collective Qi. Please note that in the Maciocia Foundations book there is a Chinese character for zong qi. My professors said this is the wrong character. I can neither confirm nor deny. I'm doing good to be speaking English and bad Spanish! I've got no Chinese.

Zong Qi is located in the chest, midway between the breasts/nips. This is where Ren 17 is, on the anterior midline, level with the 4th intercostal space. Zong Qi is clear Qi (O_2) + Gu Qi. Zong Qi therefore consists of both Wei Qi and Ying Qi living in the chest.

Zong Qi as four major functions:

1. Nourishes the Heart and Lungs

2. Runs inside the Lungs through the throat to help respiration. It also enters the Blood vessels to help the

Heart and promote Blood circulation. Together these two sub-functions bridge the Heart and Lungs.

3. Controls speech and volume of the voice.
A soft voice with shortness of breath indicates a Zong Qi deficiency. Qigong can greatly improve this.

4. Involves circulation of Blood in the extremities as well as feeling and sensation of movement in the extremities. After a stroke, a patient's Zong Qi is often blocked causing disorders in both sensation and movement.

True Qi

True Qi is also called Zhen Qi, a Daoist term which includes both Wei and Ying Qi. Some sources say it is Zong Qi plus the Yuan Qi. Some say it is the same as Zheng or Upright Qi.

Zheng Qi

Zheng Qi, or Upright Qi, includes all positive energies previously discussed including Yuan, Wei, Ying, regenerative abilities, etc. Disease is the fight between Zheng Qi and invading pathogens or evils. This is why when a person has very weak Qi there is often a lack of symptoms of a disease – because there is very little fight that can be mustered!

This explains why elderly people often do not manifest symptoms as violently as a younger basically stronger person. Urinary Tract Infections (UTIs)are an excellent example. Younger people will have the typical signs and symptoms: burning, urgency, dark urine, maybe even a fever. Older people often have zero symptoms except for the dark urine. No burning, no fevers, don't even know they have an infection until they rather suddenly get delirious, start talking trash, and make no sense. In older people, sudden onset of dementia like symptoms is often the first indication of a UTI. The same is true of pneumonia. Many times an elderly person doesn't even know they have it. They just assume they have a little cold.

Moral to the story: don't discount mild symptoms in elderly patients!

Zhong Qi

Zhong Qi (pronounced "tsong"), is also called *Central* Qi and indicates the Qi of the Spleen and Stomach, which is the place these two organs occupy (center/middle) in the Five Element Theory. Zhong Qi is thus the nickname for Spleen/Stomach Qi.

"Bu zhong yi Qi tang" is a formula from Li Dong Yuan's *Treatise on Stomach and Spleen*. Bu Zhong Yi Qi tang translates to "tonify middle, replenish Qi decoction."

GENERAL FUNCTIONS OF QI

Six general functions of Qi I'm going to need you to memorize for my non-existent quiz! But seriously, know these. I'll do them in a chart for you:

Memorize this column	A little explanation/example column that you don't need to memorize
Transformation	Yuan Qi facilitates this transformation. Yuan Qi is the building block Qi that is transformed to every other kind of Qi. *Chinese texts say this is the most important function of Qi*
Transportation	This is about the dynamic nature of Qi. When Qi stops, the body dies. Think about Spleen and Heart Qi moving Blood, Lung Qi moving the Wei Qi to the skin and spreads it out, etc.

Raising	Spleen Qi/Yang raising Qi and supporting/holding organs. Kidney Qi also has a raising function.
Warming	Body temperature is maintained by Spleen Qi, Yuan Qi from Kidney + Mingmen fire, and Wei Qi. Blood and thus Heart Qi keeps the body warm too.
Holding	Not the same as storing. Storing is accumulation with an organ. Holding is consolidation and prevention of leakage – like a dam holds water. Examples: <ul><li>Lung Qi problems can = nasal discharge.</li><li>Heart Qi deficiency can = profuse sweating</li><li>Kidney Qi deficiency can = urinary or stool incontinence, premature ejaculation, profuse vaginal discharge.</li><li>Spleen Qi deficiency can = drooling, Blood vessel leakage (Spleen holds the Blood in the vessels)</li><li>Liver Qi stagnation can = weeping, crying, depression</li></ul>
Protecting	All internal organ Qi has a protective function. Wei and Zheng/Upright Qi, for example.

MOVEMENT OF QI AND DIRECTION OF QI FLOW IN THE ZANGFU

Qi moves through the channels in a circular motion without ceasing. There are four forms of this Qi movement.

Direction	Explanation
Ascending	Also called upward going or upgoing in some literature. Qi lifts.
Descending	Also written as downward going and downgoing. Qi desends.
Entering	Also = ingoing and inward going. Entering the body, in other words.
Exiting	Also called outgoing, spreading, and dispersing. Refers to it exiting one place in the body and moving or dispersing to other places.

Different organs have different directional flows and therefore different functions in the body. And once again, Maciocia's book is going to disagree with what I say here, but I'm listening to the Chinese doctors from China, most of whom have been studying this for the last 40-60 years.

Note that *all* of the Yang organs have a descending function and also note that the most important directional flows are below in red.

Zang	Qi direction/s	Fu	Qi direction/s
Lung (LU)	All 4 directions: • Ascend = exhale • Descending for various functions • Disperse/exiting for various functions • Entering/ingoing = inhale	Large Intestine (LI or CO)	Descending *(CO = colon, fyi)*
Heart (HT)	• Exiting = pumping of Blood – disperses it to all parts • Descending via channel connection to SI (Small intestine) • Ascending. Channel connects to eyes, HT condition shows in complexion	Small Intestine (SI)	Descending
Spleen (SP)	• Ascending. Channel originates at great toe, terminates at the root of the tongue. Also has the function of ascending clear Yang.	Stomach (ST)	Descending When it doesn't there is food stagnation, belching, nausea, vomiting, etc. Qi going the wrong direction.

Liver (LV or LR)	• Ascending. • Exiting. Spreading of the Liver Qi. No exiting = Liver Qi stagnation.	Gallbladder (GB)	Descending
Kidney (KD)	• Ascending • Descending • Entering - ingoing	Urinary Bladder (BL or UB)	Descending
Pericardium (PC)	• Entering • Exiting	San Jiao (SJ, TB, TW)	• Ascending • Descending

I've paired the Zang and Fu organs across the row in this table. Note the abbreviations under each organ name. You'll see these over and over again. Might as well get used to them now.

Final note about the chart: San Jiao has to both ascend and descend since it is the water moving system of the body.

PATHOLOGIES OF QI

There are two main parts to this discussion, which is a lengthy one.

First, we will discuss the disorder of the amount or volume of qi. There can be either too much or too little. If there is too much qi, there is fire in the body. An example is Heart fire, a hyperfunctioning of Heart Qi in which there is too much. There can also be too little Qi resulting in a Qi deficiency pattern or syndrome.

Second, we will discuss *disorders* of Qi movement. Here are the ones to know. *All* Qi pathologies fall into these categories in some manner. We will discuss these in further detail below.

Pathology of Qi	Quick explanation
Qi deficiency	Not enough or poor quality. All organs can have Qi deficiency except the Liver.
Qi stagnation	Movement of Qi from all directions slows down. . . so does everything else associated with it.
Qi rebellion	Too much Qi ascending or going the wrong direction.

Qi prolapse syndrome	Qi descends too much (or just can't lift resulting in falling) eventually causing organ prolapse
Qi closing syndrome	Aka, Qi tense syndrome
Qi collapsing syndrome	Results in death.

A couple of things to know about the discussion below.

- Your patients won't necessarily have *all* of the signs and symptoms listed, but will often have several at a time.

- Patients have more than just one thing going on at a time. You'll see other symptoms and signs mixed in. Your job is to add up the clues you see.

- **Memorize *all* of these syndromes and signs/symptoms.** You'll see them all over just about every test you will take in regards to Chinese medicine.

- Finally, the difference between signs and symptoms:
  o *Signs are objective.*
    You as the practitioner can detect them easily – pulses, facial complexions, temperature of the skin, how the tongue looks….those are signs.
  o *Symptoms are subjective.*
    Only the subject (your patient) can tell you about them because you can't detect them. Nausea, itching, and even palpitations are symptoms.
  o Signs and symptoms are often abbreviated as S/SX or s/sx…which I will likely do below.

Qi Deficiency Syndrome

All organs *except the Liver* can suffer from a Qi deficiency, but it is most likely to happen to these organs in this order: Lung, Spleen, Kidney, and Heart. Different organs will express different symptoms *in combination with these general* Qi Deficiency Syndrome symptoms:

General s/sx of a Qi deficiency

S/sx	Brief discussion
Fatigue, low energy level, tiredness, exhaustion	Qi feeds and energizes the body. Depletion of Qi gives these sensations.
Pale complexion	Can also be a sign of Blood deficiency. Make sure all of the s/sx add up to Qi deficiency.
Tongue: could be normal size, swollen, swollen with teeth marks	Tongue presentation will depend upon organ/s affected
Pulse: deep and weak	Deep pulse can also be sign of Blood deficiency, but will feel very thin from the left to the right sides of the vessel.

Lung Qi deficiency

You will see all or some of the *general* s/sx, but these will be in addition to that and are specific to a Lung Qi xu.

S/sx	Brief discussion
Shortness of breath (SOB)	Shortness of breath + coughing are *hallmark* s/sx of a Lung Qi deficiency.
Spontaneous sweating	Sweat *very* easily, like with no provocation. Why? Qi can't control the sweating pores on the skin, which is part of the Lung system. Insufficient Qi to generate Wei Qi, which controls the pores.
Soft, weak voice	Not enough energy to push the air through the vocal cords to make noise!
Catches cold easily	Lung governs immune function and is the first interface with the outside world. Pathogens inhaled cannot be overcome.

Spleen Qi xu

As with all of these, look for general Qi xu s/sx, but if there is a Spleen Qi xu, you'll see some or all of these as well.

S/sx	Brief discussion
Poor or no appetite	If the Spleen can't process it, it's not going to want more food.
Fullness in the abdomen	Even before or in the absence of eating. The area *wants to be touched*. When there is a deficiency this is generally true – touch feels good.
Chronic diarrhea or loose stool	S/sx may include diarrhea after eating oily or rich foods.

Kidney Qi xu

Kidney Qi xu includes general symptoms plus:

S/sx	Brief discussion
Weak and/or sore lower back	Maybe the knees too. Pretty common.
Frequent urination – profuse and clear	Have to pee a lot, not a lot of color to the urine.
Incontinence of urine and/or stool	Also a fairly common symptom. Women in menopause or after childbirth are often suffering from Kidney Qi xu and will leak urine when they laugh or cough. Also common to have a very sudden urge to pee and can't get to the bathroom fast enough.

Heart Qi xu

Heart Qi xu includes all symptoms of general Qi xu plus:

S/sx	Brief discussion
Palpitations	Landmark symptom of HT dysfunction. Palpitations are a symptom, not a sign. You as the practitioner can't feel them, but the patient can.
Poor spirit or insufficient Shen	Like a lack of motivation, for instance.

Excessive Internal Organ Fire

Liver fire, Stomach fire, and Heart fire are the most likely kinds you will see. This table contains the *general* s/sx.

S/sx	Brief discussion
Excitable emotional state	Pretty classic internal heat sign.
Irritable	

Feels hot	Heat burns off the body fluids
Thirsty for cold drinks	
Red face	Heat rising upward
Loud voice	
Dark yellow, scanty urine	Heat burning Body Fluids
Constipation	Body Fluids are needed to lubricate the intestines
Tongue: red body with a yellow coating	Heat rising to the tongue/head
Pulse: fast/rapid and/or slippery and/or forceful	Internal heat frequently looks like this in the pulse.

Liver Fire

General symptoms above plus:

S/sx	Brief discussion
Red eyes	"Like a rabbit" my professor said. My translation: red sclera, may even look reddish on the iris.
Bitter taste in the mouth	Burned flavor or bitterness that persists
Burning pain in the hypochondriac region	Hypochondria = below the rib cage
Heavy menstruation + fresh red blood	Like really profuse. Always ask about the color of the bloods. It tells you a lot
Irritability	Easy to anger or get pissed

Heart Fire

General symptoms above plus:

S/sx	Brief discussion
Tachycardia	Fast heartbeat – 90bpm and up
Manic behavior and restlessness	Energy can't settle because fire of the Ht disturbs the Blood
Insomnia	Can't get to sleep easily – see mania
Tossing and turning	In bed, obviously – see insomnia!
Tongue ulcers	Heart opens to the tongue, so inflamed places on tongue are common.
UTI like s/sx	HT can't handle fire, so hands it off to SI. SI descending energy transfers it to the BL for disposal. Unfortunately, the BL is prone to excess, so the heat gets stuck and = UTI s/sx.

Stomach Fire

General symptoms above plus:

S/sx	Brief discussion
Halitosis	Bad mouth odor.
Swelling and/or bleeding gums	ST channel opens into the mouth. Generally ST is associated with upper gums, LI with lower gums.
Acid reflux	Duh, right?
Burning pain in epigastric region	Stomach area. Pain + burning sensation.

Qi Stagnation Syndrome

This is *always* an excess. Stagnation is never a deficiency. It *can,* however result from a deficiency. Why? Because a deficiency means a condition of not enough. If there isn't enough Qi or enough energy to move, then Qi gets stuck as a result, building up behind the deficiency.

Go outside and turn on a water hose. Now pick it up anywhere in the middle and crimp it shut by folding it in half. Notice how the hose feels on the 'full' side – rigid, unsquishable. Notice how the hose feels on the other side. Hollow and floppy. You have created a stagnation on one side and a deficiency on the other.

OK, that's a good example of the combination of deficiency and excess/stagnation, but that didn't come about because of deficiency, it happened because you crimped the hose. An example in nature could be a slow moving river that builds up debris and sludge. If stuff floats lazily downstream and eventually lodges in one spot and builds up, it can impede the flow of the river. A bunch of water builds up behind the 'dam.' Now you have an example of deficiency causing stagnation.

You are likely to see Qi stagnation in the Liver, Spleen/Stomach (Middle Jiao), and Lung (emphysema is a version of this). You will *never* see Kidney Qi stagnation because it doesn't exist – Kidneys can have no excess!

General s/sx of a Qi stagnation syndrome

S/sx	Explanation
Distending, wandering pain with fullness	Pain that feels like it's too full. Pain wanders around, isn't fixed. Worse with stress and depression
Aversion to touch	Feels worse with pressure or touch. There's already too much here. Touch adds to the excess.*
Tongue body and coating could be normal	No specific "Qi stagnation" signs for tongue
Pulse is wiry or short	Wiry is a common pulse to find in Qi stagnation.

*One way you determine excess vs deficiency is by pressing – if it feels better with pressure or touch, it's probably a deficiency. If it feels worse, it's most likely an excess.

Liver Qi Stagnation

General symptoms above plus:

S/sx	Explanation
Stress and/or depression	Frequent bouts of this.
Sighing a lot	Sighs frequently. This is the body's attempt to move the Qi that gets stuck in the chest
Fullness or distention in the chest/breast area	Hence the sighing! But this can go even further than just the chest sensation. In women, this includes the fullness and distended feeling in the breasts that come with PMS and sometimes with the period.
Hypochondriac pain	You'll also see this called flank pain in some Chinese medical literature – pain on the sides of the body around the bottom and just below the rib cage.
PMS	Premenstrual syndrome
Pulse	Wiry pulse. Classic sign of Liver Qi stagnation. You might feel it on the left in the Liver pulse, but not uncommon to feel it on the right instead in the middle position where you usually find the Spleen pulse.

Middle Jiao (Spleen/Stomach) Qi Stagnation

General symptoms above plus:

S/sx	Explanation
Depressed or no appetite	There's already too much stuff stuck. Body doesn't want more!
Full feeling in the abdomen	Worse than with Qi deficiency of the Middle Jiao – and feels worse with pressing or touching.
Gas and bloating	Because the Qi can't move through to clear it
Distending pain in the abdomen	Pain associated with it feeling to full
Aversion to touch	When there is an excess the body doesn't want more. Touch and pressure adds a sensation of "more" and it feels bad.

Lung Qi Stagnation

This isn't asthma or cough. Though asthma and coughing can come from heat and phlegm or cold and phlegm, it's often a *deficient* condition at its' root. This is something different, even though some of the s/sx look asthma-like.

This is definitely an excess and is more associated with emphysema.

Look for the general symptoms of Qi stagnation plus:

S/sx	Explanation
Chest tightness	Due to the excessive Qi stuck here
Dyspnea	Difficulty breathing. Same deal – too much Qi to move here already, so it's hard to get a breath
Emphysema	Look for an enlarged, barrel chest. The Qi is stuck, so the intercostal area is distended or enlarged. An emphysema patient will often lean forward and rest their elbows on their knees, a position that takes pressure off of the chest and lets them breathe easier

Qi Rebelling Syndrome

Rebelling Qi is Qi that is either ascending too much or descending too much. When you see Qi ascending too much, you are likely to see it in the Liver and Lung. When you see Qi *descending* too much, you're likely to find it in the Lung and/or Stomach.

What are the general s/sx of a Qi Rebellion Syndrome? There aren't any. They are all organ-specific.

Lung Qi Rebelling Syndrome

S/sx	Explanation
Coughing	Qi isn't moving like it should and phlegm is getting stuck
Wheezing	Same.
Asthma	Both difficulty breathing and wheezing = asthma.
Superficial breathing	No deep breaths, dispersing function isn't really online
Tongue and pulse?	Nothing specific

Stomach Qi Rebelling Syndrome

S/sx	Explanation
Nausea	Qi isn't descending sufficiently
Vomiting	
Retching	*Retching is trying to vomit but all that*
Hiccups	*happens is dry heaves. Bummer.*
Heart burn or acid reflux	Not the burning pain of stomach fire, but probably due to food not descending to the SI because the ST Qi isn't going downward
Tongue and pulse?	Nothing specific

Liver Qi Rebelling Syndrome

S/sx	Explanation
Irritability	Liver moves Qi around the body. When its'
Anger	Qi is rebelling, the emotions take a hit.
Throbbing headache	One branch of the Liver channel goes to
Dizziness/vertigo	the top of the head. The Gallbladder channel, Lv's coupled organ/channel, goes to the temple and into the ears. Lv Qi rebelling can affect the Gb channel as well.

Qi Prolapse Syndrome

Qi Prolapse Syndrome occurs when the Qi descends either too much or not enough. This is the *opposite* of a Qi Rebellion Syndrome. When the Spleen Qi does not ascend, for instance, it does not raise the organs and results in Qi and (eventually) organ prolapse. When the Kidney ascends too little then there is also prolapse. As a matter of fact, Qi Prolapse is most often a result of Kidney and/or Spleen dysfunction.

Spleen Qi Prolapse Syndrome

Qi Prolapse is an advanced form of Qi deficiency. Organ prolapse is an advanced form of both.

Remember the s/sx of Spleen Qi deficiency? Fatigue, pale face, chronic diarrhea and/or loose stool? All of those still apply. So do the general Qi deficiency s/sx. Additionally, you'll see these possible s/sx. Bu zhong Yi Qi Tang is the most commonly prescribed formula for this problem. Note the addition of the 'sinking feeling' below.

S/sx	Explanation
Sensation of fullness in lower abdomen plus a sinking sensation	Similar to the SP Qi xu/deficiency signs you saw earlier, but lower in the belly and with the sinking feeling
Hypotension	Low Blood pressure
Internal organ prolapses	Most commonly: • Stomach • Kidney • Bladder • Uterus • Anus
Pulse is deeper than with Qi xu/deficiency	The further a problem advances the deeper the pulse for it will tend to sink.

Kidney Qi Prolapse Syndrome

Like with the Spleen Qi Prolapse Syndrome, this includes Kidney Qi deficiency, just a more advanced version. You'll find all of the Qi deficiency s/sx in addition to the Kidney Qi deficiency s/sx here.

Kidney Qi deficiency s/sx included fatigue, pale face, frequent/clear/profuse urination, lower back and/or knee pain and weakness. Tongue could be pale, swollen body with teeth marks, and a white moist and wet coating. Pulse is likely to be deep and weak.

When Kidney Qi deficiency progresses to a Kidney Qi Prolapse, look for:

S/sx	Explanation
Dribbling of urine	Progressing from frequency to inability to hold
Urinary and/or stool incontinence	
Prolapse of *uterus*	More specific organ association than in Sp Qi Prolapse
Habitual miscarriage	Insufficient Ki Qi will not support a fetus
Pulse is much deeper that with Ki Qi Xu	Problem is going deeper into the body.

Qi Closing or Qi Tense Syndrome
This is an emergency situation. This might be a tonic/clonic seizure like you see in epilepsy or it could be a patient dying from toxic gas inhalation (carbon monoxide, etc.) Hopefully, this will be a rare thing for you to see.

Lung, Pericardium, and Heart are the organs that are most often affected. Because this is an emergency situation, your best treatment is to call 911. This is true for a known epileptic person too. Seizures that last for more than 5 minutes or that result in loss of consciousness can have dire consequences. If this happens on your acupuncture table, you need to find a way to get them off the table and safely onto the floor.

In ancient times Hua Tuo said to use a 3-5 cun needle to needle Ren 1. I know you don't know where Ren 1 is yet if you just started studying acupuncture, so look it up in your Deadman book (which, by the way, is totally worth having on a digital medium) and feel free to utter an expletive or three.

This probably wouldn't be a recommended treatment in this day and legal climate. Besides, we mostly have 911 now. Hua Tuo didn't really have that option.

Symptoms and signs to look for, in addition to your own self yelling, "Oh, *fxxx*!:"

S/sx	Explanation
Sudden loss of consciousness, often with falling down	I say often because epileptics sometimes have warning s/sx so they get someplace safe.
Everything is clenched	Jaw, teeth, mouth, fists. Hence the "closing " part of the name of this syndrome.
Convulsions	Part of the tight thing happening above.
Tetany and seizure	Same. What it tetany? Intermittent muscle spasms.
"Screaming like pig or sheep"	I'm not making that up. That's literally what my Chinese profs said.
Eyes rolled back in the head	"Upward staring eyes" is how you see this worded in Chinese medical literature. Eyes are rolled back in the head and all you see are the sclera.
Tongue body is stiff	Are you bloody likely to be checking for this if you are there when it happens? Probably not! You're too busy trying to dial 911.
Pulse is wiry	

Qi Collapse Syndrome

This is an emergency situation also. Look at these s/sx. Looks a helluvalot like dying, doesn't it? Call 911, will ya?

S/sx	Explanation
Loss of consciousness or semi-consciousness	The Qi is clearly collapsing in on itself here.
Pale face	
Fatigue/exhaustion	
All s/sx of Qi deficiency	

Profuse spontaneous sweating	This happens with heart attack patients too.
Leakage of body fluids	Incontinence of stool/urine, nasal discharge, saliva
Tongue has a pale swollen body and a white coating	Consistent with Blood slowing down and/or stopping. Dying people get very very pale everywhere. Even dark skinned people will look more pale and then bluish grey.
Pulse is indistinct	

And *that*, my friends is the end of Qi Chat.

CHAPTER 3
Blood

That darn Maciocia says Blood is a type of Qi. My professors disagreed and we've already talked about how I feel aout that, so….. Blood is fluid and substantive and doesn't that already sound more like yin than qi? Yeah. I rest my case.

> *"Blood is a red, fluid-like vital substance and is one of the most important in the human body."*
> — *Dr. Qianzhi Wu*

SOURCE OF BLOOD

The Spleen and Stomach are the original source of Blood. I think this might be easier to understand with a biomedical explanation with a Chinese medical explanation complement.

Biomed-speak
> You eat and drink. Your stomach grinds it all up into chyme, then sends it to your small intestine for nutrient and liquid extraction. It goes to the liver for a toxin screen and whatever is ok is passed on to the body for distribution. "Distribution" means it goes into the Blood stream as floating components headed for whatever needs it. These components are fluids, platelets, Blood cells, proteins, sugars, minerals, etc that are distributed by the Blood.

Chinesemed-speak
> You eat and drink. Stomach/Spleen take are of the digestion process and produces Ying Qi - nutritive Qi - which is sent to the Lung for distribution via its' dispersing abilities. Lung sends it to the Heart which combines Ying Qi and Body Fluids to create Blood.

The Heart gets help with this function from the Yuan Qi of the Kidneys. Biomedically speaking, you might remember that

Blood is made in the bone marrow. Kidney's relation to bone and marrow in TCM is a reflection on this.

So the organs involved in the creation of Blood are:
- Spleen and Stomach (Middle Jiao)
- Lungs
- Heart
- Kidney (Yuan Qi)

FUNCTIONS OF BLOOD

Blood has three basic functions:

Nourish the physical body	Blood is closely related to Ying Qi, which nourishes and has the function of transforming Blood.
Moistens the tissues	Blood is related to Body Fluids also which nourish and moisten the body tissues
Blood is the material foundation of Shen	This includes memory, concentration, thinking, intelligence. Blood is specifically related to short term memory. A Blood deficiency induces Shen problems as well as poor short term memory and concentration. Anemia often does this too as does a hypo-active thyroid. Yin and Blood deficiencies are more difficult to treat than yang and Qi deficiencies.

RELATIONSHIP OF BLOOD TO INTERNAL ORGANS

This is a bit of a review. Remember the Zangfu discussions from the first book (*Chinese Medicine 101: Start with the Foundations*, available on Amazon in both digital and print formats) – Heart, Spleen, and Liver are closely related to the Blood.

Organ	Ways in which it interacts with Blood
Heart	Transforms (creates) and transports (pumps) Blood. Controls the blood vessels. To nourish Blood, tonify Heart Qi. Irregular pulse can indicate Heart dysfunction.
Spleen	Generates and produces Blood. Holds it in the vessels, prevents leaking and bleeding.

Liver	Stores Blood, regulates its' distribution. Some Liver dysfunctions in Chinese medicine can cause an elevation in blood pressure.*
Lungs	"Control the 100 Vessels." Flow of Blood is related to Lung function – helps Blood to flow, adjusts the rhythm of the flow, makes it flow in waves. Slow the breath and can slow the heartbeat too. Lung cleanses and regenerates Blood. . . but does *not produce Blood.*
Kidney	Not directly involved in transformation and transport of Blood, but in an emergency situation Kidney essence is said to be converted into blood. In biomedicine we know that blood volume is controlled by the kidneys.*

*Blood pressure is largely determined by the condition of the blood vessels (whether pliable and clean, constricted by stress or pain, stiff and blocked, etc) and the blood volume.

In the clinic you will see differentiations of Heart Blood Deficiency (also called Heart Xue Xu) and Liver Blood Deficiency (Liver Xue Xu), but never Spleen Blood Deficiency since Spleen is the source of Blood.

RELATIONSHIP OF QI AND BLOOD

Qi to Blood

Qi is said to be the "Commander of the Blood." Thus, if one has a Qi and Blood deficiency, tonify the Qi first which will then nourish the Blood. Qi is far easier to treat than Blood and it responds faster. Additionally, Blood cannot recover without strong Qi.

Qi generates Blood	Via the Ying Qi, Spleen Qi, and Heart Qi
Qi moves Blood	With the Heart Qi
Qi holds Blood	This is Spleen Qi's function

Blood to Qi

Blood roots and holds Qi	It is the dense material and environment that gives Qi a home base.
Nourishes Qi	Qi nourishes Blood and Blood nourishes Qi.

RELATIONSHIP BETWEEN BLOOD AND ESSENCE

Blood and essence mutually assist each other. Here's why/how:

- When Blood is sufficient it can be transformed into acquired essence to support and assist congenital essence.

- In emergency situations, however, Kidney essence can transform directly into Blood.

Liver stores Blood while the Kidney stores Essence. The close relationship between Blood and Essence is part of the reason that Liver and Kidney have such a close relationship to each other.

PATHOLOGIES OF BLOOD

There are three syndrome disorders of Blood:
- Blood Xu Syndrome
- Blood Heat Syndrome
- Blood Stagnation Syndrome

I'll break them down for you below.

Blood Xu (deficiency) Syndrome

This refers to an *insufficient volume* of Blood. This condition affects *only* the Heart and Liver.

There are some general Blood deficiency symptoms to know and then some Heart and Liver specific ones.

General Blood Xu S/Sx

S/sx	Brief discussion
Pale or sallow face w/o luster	You need blood to bring color and warmth to the skin.
Fatigue and exhaustion	Insufficient volume and nutrients in the Blood mean your tissues aren't fed and you are easily tired
Tongue: pale, small, thin body with a normal or thin white coating	When your blood is poor either in quality or volume it cannot nourish the tongue. The thin body and paleness are the giveaways
Pulse: thin and thready	This is due to low Blood volume. This means the pulse from one side of the vessel to the other. Literally feels like your fingertips are on a thread or thin cord instead of on a full blood vessel.

Heart Blood Xu

Look for general s/sx above plus:

S/sx	Brief discussion
Palpitations	This is a subjective feeling – usually felt in the chest or the throat. When your patient reports this, start looking for Ht related things.
Dream disturbed sleep	Often abbreviated DDS in charts. Insufficient blood volume or quality means the Shen has nowhere to rest at night so it 'invents things' in your head. That'll show ya!
Poor memory and concentration	Especially short term memory, inability to concentrate. A friend calls this "hummingbird" mind.
Pulse – like general sx	Could also be irregular, but not especially.

Liver Blood Xu

Look for general s/sx above plus:

S/sx	Brief discussion
Blurred vision, floaters, eye spots	Blurred vision despite glasses or contacts. Floaters are little black spots one can see in their field of vision when they look at a blue sky or a white background.
Numbness of extremities	Indicates lack of proper blood flow
Insomnia	This is because a lack of blood volume means insufficient Blood for the Shen to feel at home
Menstruation that is scanty, pale in color, or loose and watery	Scanty = very light periods. Pale, loose, watery = color that looks more like watercolor than Blood
Pale nails	Again, insufficient blood flow to color the skin beneath the nails
Pulse = thin, thread, wiry	Thin and thread means how it feels from one side of the blood vessel to the other under your fingertips. Wiry because that's a pulse that is often associated with Liver dysfunction.

Blood Heat Syndrome

Heat in the Blood means just what it sounds like: the Blood is literally hotter than it should be for health. I can't think of a biomedical equivalent concept for this, but it's definitely a thing.

The s/sx are divided into 2 groups: Heat s/sx and bleeding s/sx.

Blood Heat S/Sx

The general s/sx are as follows:

S/sx	Brief discussion
Red face	Heat rising to the face and showing in the
Red eyes	complexion
Thirst for cold drinks	Heat is burning off Body Fluids, causing dehydration
Constipation	Heat burning off Body Fluids in the intestine
Pulse that is fast or rapid	

Liver Blood Heat

If the heat in the blood is mainly affecting Liver Blood, the s/sx above plus:

S/sx	Brief discussion
Irritation and anger	This is Blood heat affecting the Shen

Heart Blood Heat

If heat in the blood is mainly affecting the Heart Blood, the s/sx above plus:

S/sx	Brief discussion
Tachycardia	Like a super fast pulse. 90bpm and up.
Yellow tongue coating	Yellow tongue coatings are a sign of heat somewhere in the body. You have to add up the signs and symptoms to make sure about that and to find out what kind of heat it is and what it is affecting.

Bleeding Symptoms

Heat makes the Blood flow more and faster. You will often see this called "reckless bleeding." Reckless bleeding tends to be acute (very sudden onset) and excessive.

Bleeding

This is a spontaneous bleeding, mostly in the upper part of the body. This can be epistaxis (nose bleeds) or coughing with fresh looking red blood. Blood looks bright red, will feel hot and sticky to the patient and is hard to stop. Very lava-like! That indicates an excess condition – look at all the "too much" quality here!

Dermatitis

Skin rashes? Seriously? Yes. Seriously. Skin rashes like psoriasis and other unexplained skin itching and welting with a lot of scratching and bleeding from the scratching are often driven by Blood Heat. Is it always? No. You have to add up all the s/sx to confirm that. But it happens frequently enough with this pathology that it's definitely worth knowing.

Blood Stagnation (Xue Yu) and Blood Stasis (Yu Xue)

Are you tired of typing or writing out "s-t-a-g-n-a-t-i-o-n" yet? Use the Chinese pinyin word "yu" which means "stagnation." And by the way, it's faster to write xue, the Chinese word for Blood than it is to write out Blood.

This concept is true both in biomedicine and in Chinese medicine. When the blood in the body is flowing in the usually happy manner, all is well. When blood flow slows down or gets sluggish for whatever reason, the thick and sticky components of the blood become more pronounced. They will eventually get clumpy and then clot in the vessels. This might happen because of a fibrillation problem in the heart that doesn't move the blood through properly, or because of arterial scarring and plaque buildup, or because of a clotting disorder, or because there's not sufficient "thinners" in the blood to keep it from being thick.

Regardless of the reason, Blood that slows down and get sluggish is referred to in Chinese medicine as **Blood Stagnation**. Blood is in a process of getting sluggish. Eventually, this process can result in a complete stoppage of the flow of Blood and that is called **Blood Stasis**. Blood Stasis is the result of the stagnation and that's what leads to clotting in the vessels, in the menses, and even in thrombosis leading to a stroke.

Both Blood Stagnation and Blood Stasis cause the problem of Blood not being able to flow to, feed the tissues properly, or carry waste away. The symptoms of both of these pathologies are the same. Here's what you need to know.

S/sx	Brief discussion
Pain	
• Needling or pricking pain	Tissues aren't being fed by blood, causes pain
• Fixed, not moving	Indicates the blood flow is stopped or insufficient in some area
• Aversion to touch	This is an excess – adding more with touch feels bad
• Worse at night	Blood is yin and the night is the time for yin. Makes the pain more noticeable at night.
Mass	Palpable under the skin – this could be tumor related (and tumors are often Blood Stasis related), but could also be post surgical or post injury. To help treat a mass, first send your patient to the oncologist! When you confirm it's not cancer, promote Blood flow.
Bruise	Bruises are a form of Blood Stasis. These occur after injuries – car accidents, sprained ankles, etc. Promote Blood flow to help them heal.

Irregular menstrual bleeding	Dark red to brown in color with clotting – larger than dime sized – with cramping in the abdomen.
Rough, thick, dry, dark, scaly skin	This is not always true and is less common than other s/sx
Thirsty, but doesn't want to drink	This is a less common s/sx too. Thirsty, but just wants to rinse their mouth out usually. More common in Blood Stagnation syndromes.
Pulse is hesitant or choppy, wiry, knotted	Knotted is a slow pulse, less than 60bpm and is irregular. You'll learn more about the pulse types later in Diagnostics studies.
Tongue* <ul><li>Purple body</li><li>Purple spots on tongue</li></ul>	Purple body because lack of proper blood flow Not where the spots are on the tongue. The location can tell you what organ is likely affected. You'll learn more about this in Diagnostics studies.

This page intentionally left blank.

CHAPTER 4
Body Fluids

Body Fluid is a fluid-like vital substance which contains *jin* (associated with Wei Qi) and *ye* (associated with Ying Qi). The source of fluids in the body are the Spleen, Stomach, Small Intestine and Large Intestine. What I mean by that is that these four organs generate and transform Body Fluids. Body Fluids must be transported through the body and discharged/excreted as needed.

Transportation of body fluids

Three organs are responsible for transportation of body fluids are:

Lung	Upper Jiao
Spleen	Middle Jiao
Kidney	Lower Jiao

Of the three, Spleen is the most important for transportation and works as a pivot between the Upper and Lower Jiao. Here is why:

- Spleen Qi generates Lung Qi.
  Looking at it from Five Element theory, Spleen (Earth) is the Mother of Lung (Metal). Because Earth generates Metal, all Lung functions rely on the Spleen.

- Spleen controls the Kidney
  This is another five element relationship: earth controlling water.

Discharge and excretion of Body Fluids

Two organs are "on call" when the body neds to discharge or excrete Body Fluids: Lung and Kidney.

Kidneys

You could make an argument for including the yang organs of the Bladder and Large Intestine, but Kidney controls the opening and closing of both the urethra and the anal opening regardless. And besides they're paired with those yin organs anyhow).

Lung

The Lung controls sweating and opens the sweating pores to release body fluids. The Lung also breathes out vapor. Kidney controls urination. Of the two organs, Kidney is the more important one in this function as it is able to discharge about three times more waste from the body than the Lung does.

RELATIONSHIP OF THE BODY FLUIDS WITH THE INTERNAL ORGANS

We're bags of mostly water, but it's still worth knowing which organs have what relationship with the Body Fluids and how that relationship goes down. Spleen, Lung, and Kidney are the 3 most directly involved organs in body fluid metabolism because they directly influence water metabolism, so let's start with them.

Yin Organ	Primary Function	Explanation/discussion
Spleen	Transformation Transportation	Most important organ for transformation and transportation of Body Fluids. But it does not involve the excretion of fluids. Because of Spleen's position in the Middle Jiao, it has no connection to the orifices or pores.
Lungs	Transportation Excretion Regulate water passages	Lungs complete these functions using the water passages of the San Jiao channel. The controls the distribution of body fluids depending on the temperature, etc. It does not, however, involve the *generation* of water or body fluids. In *The Golden Chamber* Zhang Zhongjing said that edema above the waist is largely a dysfunction of the

		Lung. To resolve upper body edema, promote sweating with herbs such as Ma Huang.
Kidneys	Transportation of Body Fluids	Kidney Yang steams Body Fluids up to the Lung, which disperses them "like a fine mist" through the body, says Chinese medical literature.
	Excretion	Kidney controls the opening and closing of the Bladder to release fluid wastes. In *The Golden Chamber* Zhang Zhongjing said that edema below the waist is largely a dysfunction of the Kidney. Resolve edema in the lower body by promoting urination with herbs having a diuretic function.
	Transformation	Kidney Qi and Yang support, facilitate, and transform Body Fluids indirectly through supporting the Spleen, Large Intestine, Small Intestine and Stomach. Kidneys are the lower *source* and *container* (in the Lower Jiao) of fluids in the body.

Now let's look at the three corresponding yang/Fu organs' role in body fluids.

Yang Organ	Primary Function	Explanation/discussion
Urinary Bladder	Holding Excretion	When what biomedicine calls "urine" is in the BL is still considered to be Body Fluids until it is released from the body. Kidney controls the opening and closing of the Bladder orifice.

San Jiao	Transportation	It is the Yang water passage organ throughout the trunk. Does not directly excrete or transform.
Stomach	Transformation Generation	You eat and drink it, the Stomach grinds it up and gives it to the Spleen.

RELATIONSHIP OF QI AND BODY FLUID

This is the basically the same relationship structure as you found in the Blood and Qi section in the previous chapter.

Qi to Body Fluids

Qi generates/produces Body Fluids	Unless there is insufficient intake to do so.
Qi moves/transports Body Fluids	Unless there is retention or stagnation of fluids
Qi holds Body Fluids	Unless there is leakage such as spontaneous sweating, frequent urination or urinary incontinence

Body Fluids to Qi

Body Fluid carries Qi	Carries it through the whole body. Dehydration results in a loss of fluids, but also a loss of Qi....which is why fatigue accompanies dehydration.
	Best herb for this? American ginseng (or Xi Yang Shen), which nourishes fluids, tonifies Qi.
	Tonify Qi to help generate fluids.

RELATIONSHIP OF BLOOD AND BODY FLUID

Blood and Body Fluid derive from the same source, Stomach and Spleen. They are also mutually supportive. When one thrives, so does the other. When one is weak, so is the other.

Blood and Body fluid derive from the same source	Spleen and Stomach. If there is enough Blood, there is enough Body Fluid
Blood and Body fluid are mutually supported	Body fluid flows outside the vessels while Blood flows within them. In Chinese medicine they are considered the same fluid, only varying by location. • If Blood is deficient, Body Fluids from soft tissues can go into the vessels to supplement Blood. • If Body Fluids are deficient, Blood will compensate in a similar manner.

Important Clinical Principles

Now that you know the chart above, this should make sense. Keep these principles in mind when you go into clinic to observe or when you begin to treat.

Blood Deficient patients	Never promote sweating in Blood deficient patients. This is contraindicated. Sweating will further deplete Blood, which will try to compensate for lost fluids and get even more deficient.
Body Fluid Deficient patients	Do not promote circulation of Body Fluids and be very careful about promoting Blood circulation, as this can cause more deficiency.

RELATIONSHIP OF ESSENCE AND BODY FLUID

Don't worry about it. It's not a "thing," so there's nothing to know.

DIFFERENCE BETWEEN JIN AND YE

These flow in the Body Fluids. Be aware of the differences between them.

Jin	Ye
Light, watery, clear type of Body Fluid	Heavy, sticky, turbid part of Body Fluid
Example: tears, saliva	Example: CSF, synovial fluid
Superficial, runs with the Wei Qi	Localized, runs deeper, moves with the Ying Qi
Quicker, more generalized	Slower, more static/localized
Easily nourished	Hard to nourish
More Yang	More Yin

FUNCTION OF BODY FLUIDS

- Moisten the tissues
  Both the jin and ye do this, but jin moreso.

- Nourish the body
  This is more of a ye function. Ye is heavy and sticky, similar to ying qi.

- Body fluids are part of the blood.

There are two patterns (deficiency and retention) and four syndromes (Body Fluid Deficiency, Damp Retention, Phlegm Retention, and Water Retention).

Body Fluid Deficiency

Body Fluid deficiency is a pathology that primarily affects the Lung, Stomach and Large Intestine (but *never* the Liver, Heart or Spleen). The best treatment is dietary supplements and herbs, which work better than acupuncture for this problem.

General Symptoms

Dryness	Of mouth, skin, hair, lips, and stool. Very likely scanty urine too.
Tongue	Body is small and thin, color is normal. Coat is rough, dry, normal color.
Pulse	Thin and thready

Body Fluid Deficiency affecting Lung

General s/sx plus:

Cough	Dry with no mucus or little mucus that is hard to expel
Nose	Dry with itching

Body Fluid Deficiency affecting Stomach

General s/sx plus:

Pain	Burning pain in epigastric region
Thirst	With desire to drink
Retching	Dry heaves, ya know?
Tongue	Dry with cracks, mirror or no coating.

Body Fluid Deficiency affecting Large Intestine

General s/sx plus:

Stool	Constipation and/or dry stool
Urine	Scanty

Retention of Body Fluids

Retention of Body fluids is a pathology that causes a retention (an excess) of Damp. Damp retention results from Spleen dysfunction, impairing Spleen's ability to transport water. Damp retention is the most basic of Body Fluid retentions.

Phlegm Retention ◄——— Heated by LU or ST heat ——— Dampness (Spleen) ——— Cooled by SP or KI Yang Xu ——► Water Retention

Dampness + Heat = Phlegm Retention

Damp is 'cooked' by heat into a thicker form of Damp - Phlegm. You do something similar in cooking when you make a reduction by simmering away liquids to make a thick sauce.

Smoking tobacco or any other herb adds fire directly to the Lung, causing mucus (which is usually worse in the mornings).

Spicy, fried and grilled food causes more fire in the body also. Cooking by frying and grilling adds even more fire quality to food. The food retains this property whether it is *physically* hot when you eat it or not.

Phlegm in the Lung tends to go upward, as it is the lung's job to expel extra Phlegm.

Damp + Cold = Water Retention

The problem here is *insufficient warmth* to keep the dampness from congealing. If you've ever made ice cream or frozen yogurt you have used this principle to change liquids to solids by applying cold. Insufficient warmth also keeps the body from moving the water properly.

Consumption of dairy products (milks, cheeses , ice cream, creamers, etc – especially cow dairy products), foods with cold properties (seafoods, seaweeds, watermelon, tofu) will all cause more damp and cold in the body, making this problem worse.

Retention of water tends to go *downward* in the body, collecting most noticeably in the lower extremities.

"Spleen is the source of phlegm while Lungs store the phlegm."

Section 2: Organ Relationships and Interactions

This is a brief introduction to the ten inter-relationships between the Yin/Zang organs and how they interact with Essence, Qi, Blood, Body Fluids, etc. You'll get far more of this in Diagnostics texts, but this is a nice soft intro for you for now. There is a very short section on Yang relationships, but that's pretty simple and easy.

Even though it's just a brief introduction, you'll do well to pack this into your head now so that when you get to Diagnostics it feels more familiar.

> You have to know the organ functions to understand how they interact together. Once you know that, you can understand the interactions between the organs.
>
> The interactions are very important and in some cases more important than the individual functions!

Now onward with the inevitable charts and tables! I admit I'm a bit addicted to them.

This page intentionally left blank

CHAPTER 5
Heart Relationships

The heart in TCM holds the position of Monarch or King. All other organs support the monarch. The Lung surrounds the Heart and is regarded as the Prime Minister in Chinese medicine. Remember that the Heart transforms the Blood while the Lungs disperse, control respiration, and govern Qi.

The relationship of Heart and Lung is one of Qi and Blood and is connected by the Zong Qi.

Qi and Blood

The generation and regulation of Qi primarily involves the Lung, Liver, and Spleen.

Organ	What it does – a review
Heart	Generation of and regulation of Blood
Lung	Governs the flow of Blood through the vessels
Liver	Stores Blood
Spleen	Generates Blood, controls the flow by supplying Qi to the Heart to push the Blood through the vessels

Here's an example as to how they interact. Cigarette smoking often leads to cardiopulmonary disease. The major symptoms are:

S/sx	Explanation
Cough	The cough results from disturbed Lung Qi, affecting Qi circulation. This affects the circulation of Qi, which then affects circulation of Blood. That then impacts the Heart.
Enlarged or barrel chest	
Congestive Heart Failure	Where you see Qi deficiency, you also see Blood problems too. Thus, breath and Blood problems are linked together.

Remember that bit about Qi transforming into Blood in previous chapters? That comes into play here too. Remember too that Zong Qi is composed of Food Qi + Air Qi and resides in the chest. Long term smoking disturbs the Qi to the point that Zong Qi is weakened. Since Zong Qi assists respiration and blood circulation, it has a strong connection the Heart and Lung.

And while we're on the topic, speech and voice are good indicators of the health of the Zong Qi.

HEART AND SPLEEN

This is a relationship of Blood. In Five Element theory, this is Heart/Fire generating Spleen/Earth.

Heart (Fire)	Spleen (Earth)
Transforms Blood – transforms the components given by Spleen into Blood	Generates Blood – supplies the substantive source of Blood to the Heart
Moves/pushes the Blood through the vessels	Holds the Blood in the vessels, keeping from leaking out.

Deficiency of Heart and Spleen is a very specific pattern in TCM and is a combination of Spleen Qi Xu (deficiency) and Heart Blood Xu. The most prevalent symptom of this diagnosis is insomnia. Know why? Because a Heart Blood xu is due to a Heart Yin xu. Remember that Yin is the basis for Blood. A Heart Yin xu causes a relative increase in Heart Yang and that kind of heat disturbs the Blood causing the insomnia.

This is primarily a *Blood* relationship affecting the areas of emotions and Shen. If you look at it from a Five Element perspective, this is a control relationship with Heart/Fire controlling Lung/Metal.

Heart (Fire)	Lung (Metal)
• Moves Blood	• Stores Blood
	• Regulates flow of Blood by regulating flow of Qi
• Shen resides in the Heart, is rooted in Blood.	• Liver controls flow of Qi and thus of the flow of emotions.
When Heart is out of balance, s/sx can =	When Liver is out of balance (i.e., diagnosis of Liver Qi stagnation), s/sx can =
• Poor short term memory • Difficulty concentrating • Excess joy (think mania) • Restlessness	• Anxiety • Depression • Anger • Irritation

Think about what happens when you get super angry: blood pounds through your vessels as your heart rate increases and it's hard to think about anything other than what you are angry about.

HEART AND KIDNEY

This is the relationship between fire (Heart) and water (Kidney). This is a *circulation* relationship.
You must have a balance between the extremes of fire and water in order to function properly.

There are many references in Chinese folk tales and in Chinese literature about the fire dragon who lives deep in the sea. When water is sufficient, the dragon is calm. Without sufficient water, the dragon becomes angry and restless, taking to the skies, breathing fire and causing drought.

They must be in balance or the earth suffers. If the fire dragon prevails, the land is parched and dry. If the water dragon prevails, the land is flooded and rained out. Because the human body is an extension and part of the earth, the same applies.

When HT/KI are balanced:	Water from KI is steamed by KI Yang. Steam rises to LU and is then dispersed by the LU in a fine mist, which moistens and cools the fire of the HT. HT Yang and fire then assist KI Yang in steaming water of KI and the cycle continues like that.

When the HT/KI balance is broken:	• When KI is deficient, there is insufficient water to cool HT fire.
	S/sx =HT fire. Mental restlessness, insomnia, red face, thirst.
	
	• When the HT and KI Yin are both deficient this is called "Heart Kidney Disharmony." S/sx=
	  o Palpitations (HT)
	  o Insomnia (Blood Xu). Blood xu results from too much heat burning Body Fluids and thus too little water to create Blood, too little Yin to create the right conditions.
	  o Restless and irritability (HT fire)
	  o Poor memory/concentration (HT and KI – HT = short term memory, KI = long term memory)
	
	• Deficient HT fire or HT Yin results in too little fire to keep the water of the Kidney in balance. Too much water in the body, edema, fluid retention.
	
	• Deficient KI fire/Yin = water not steamed upward for circulation, too much water in the lower body, edema, fluid retention.

CHAPTER 6
Lung Relationships

We've already talked about Heart and Lung, so we'll skip that. As a matter of fact, these chapters will get shorter and shorter because a lot of the material on inter-relationships of the Yin organs will have been covered already.

LUNG AND LIVER

This is a Five Element relationship of Wood to Metal. This is a relationship about Qi Transformation.

Lung (Wood)	Liver (Metal)
Governs Qi and descends Qi	Ascends Qi, spreads it out in all directions (think of a tree trunk raising up into branches)
In Upper Jiao and on the right	In the Lower Jiao and on the left
Commander of the Blood vessels	Stores Blood

People with a Qi and Blood disorder have a Lung and Liver problem. Coughing blood, for example, can be a sign of Lung-Liver disharmony in which the fire of the Liver damages the Lung, causing bleeding. To stop this kind of cough, an excess, soothe/sedate the Liver (Wood) which will calm the disturbed Lung (Metal) Qi. This is Wood insulting Metal.

One more tidbit: because of the side oriented nature of these two, if you see s/sx primarily on the left, suspect Liver involvement. If you see mostly s/sx on the right, explore Lung involvement.

LUNG AND SPLEEN

This is a relationship of Qi and Body Fluid. In Five Element Speak, the element of Spleen (Earth) *generates* the element of Metal (Lung). Let's do a "line item" comparison to see how they interact.

I'm putting the Spleen in the 'beginning' column since its' element is the generator of metal. It just flows better that way. You can flip it around when you teach it to yourself if you want. Still works.

Spleen (Earth)	Lung (Metal)
Source of Blood and Qi (including LU Qi)	Controls the Qi
Helps you acquire new Qi through eating and drinking	Helps you acquire new Qi through breathing
Middle source of water (Middle Jiao)	Upper source of water (Upper Jiao)
Send water (and Qi) upward to Lung	Lung disperses water from Middle Jiao downward in a "fine mist"

If a patient has a water metabolism disorder one dysfunctional possibility is that some of the water stays in the Lung. There is a saying from the *Neijing*: "Spleen generates Phlegm. Lung stores it." What that means is that the water (the building blocks for Phlegm, if you will) comes from the Spleen, gets stuck in the Lung and then coagulates into Phlegm. Then it hangs out in the Lung until you can resolve it.

If a patient that has a lot of Phlegm and an acute problem, treat the Phlegm in the Lung. You have to figure out if it's been coagulated by cold or by heat, but you still treat it here. If this is a chronic problem that has persisted, you know that the Spleen is the root of the problem.

This is a relationship of water metabolism, of respiration, and of Qi transformation. Lung controls the breath, Kidney *roots* the breath. In Five Element Speak, that's a relationship between Metal (Lung) and Water (Kidney). Metal is then the 'mother' of Kidney.

Lung (Metal)	Kidney (Water)
Upper source (Upper Jiao) of water	Lower source (Lower Jiao) of water
Transforms Clear/Da Qi of the breath	Transforms Primary Qi
Controls the breath	Roots the breath
Disperses water down into the body in a 'fine mist.'	Kidney yang heats, recirculates the water upward in a vapor to the Upper Jiao/Lung/Heart.
Deficient Lung Qi = can't control water either of the sweating pores or the urine	Deficient Kidney Qi = can't control the lower 2 openings (anus/urethra)
Excrete water through sweat	Excrete water through the lower two openings

Some notes on the fluid metabolism relationship

The conduits for water in the body, the 'pipelines,' are the San Jiao/Triple Burner/Triple warmer.The *Neijing* says the Body Fluids are dispersed under the skin, "above" the Zangfu Organs.

There are two secretions/excretions in the body that have to do with water too: sweat and urine. When Lung Qi is deficient, one of the possible problems is that the Lung Qi cannot hold the water. When there is a deficiency of Lung Yin, people will have night sweats, usually in the upper body and chest area. If you see edema in the body, you tonify the Lung and Kidney Yang so that you can regulate this fluid metabolism thing.

Some notes on the respiration relationship

The Kidney pulls Qi from breath downward for the Lung and roots it. When the Lung holds air in, the Kidney roots this air, sucking it downward into the body like a vacuum. Shallow breathing disturbs Kidney Qi and disturbed or weakened Kidney Qi results in shallow breathing.

What did I just describe here? *One* kind of asthma. When asthma is acute and attacking actively, focus treatment on the Lung. When the patient *isn't* having an asthma attack, they are in a more chronic state, so the treatment would be tonify the Kidney, thus increasing the ability of the Kidney to root the Lung.

(Note: Maciocia discusses at least 2 types of asthma – the deficiency kinds as described here and an allergic kinds…be sure you get the types right and never assume you know the answer before all the facts have been gathered!)

CHAPTER 7
Liver Relationships

Look back at the previous chapters to see the other Liver relationships.

LIVER AND SPLEEN

This pattern combination is frequently seen in clinic. This relationship that affects both Blood and digestion. Five 'elementally,' this is a relationship between Wood and Earth.

Liver (Wood)	Spleen (Earth)
Stores Blood	Generates Blood
Responsible for the smooth flow of Qi	Generates Qi

Liver is responsible for the smooth flow of Qi and stores Blood. Spleen generates Qi *and* blood as well as holding the blood in the vessels. Spleen is the source of blood. Together, Liver and Spleen can prevent bleeding.

Digestion is another area in which Liver and Spleen must coordinate. The Spleen (yin) moves Qi upwards while the Stomach (yang) descends Qi. If the Liver overacts on the Spleen the result is Qi, which will not ascend causing diarrhea or loose stool or constipation. These will probably alternate. This is a disturbed Middle Jiao caused by Liver overacting on Spleen. Congested Liver Qi will also disturb the bile secretions.

In an ideal situation, Liver should ascend, assisting Spleen Qi.

LIVER AND KIDNEY

Liver and Kidney is a mutually beneficial relationship between Blood and Essence. It's also a relationship around storage.

Liver (Wood)	Kidney (Water)
Stores Blood	Stores Essence

The Liver stores Blood while the Kidney stores Essence. The Neijing says, "Essence and Blood have the same source." Essence is responsible for growth, development and reproduction. It also produces marrow, is the basis for Kidney Qi, and of constitutional strength. If you tonify Essence you also tonify Blood.

One example of the relationship between Kidney and Liver is aplastic anemia which is a disease of the marrow not producing Blood properly. Hypertension is also related to both Liver and Kidney. Hypertension is a classic disease of both Liver and Kidney. One form of hypertension can be a case too much Yang, for example, and occurs when Liver fire is in excess. A Kidney and Liver Yin deficiency caused by any burning or consumption of Yin, (for instance eating hot and spicy foods, many activities at night rather than sleeping, etc) will cause Yin to become less and Yang to get too strong. This causes a condition of internal wind which causes the Yang to rise in the body generating the hypertension. This can also result in dizziness and vertigo.

Think about a tornado or a hurricane: heat fronts tend to cause them causing strong wind which spirals upward. That's a parallel between the environment and our bodies.

CHAPTER 8
Spleen Relationships

Where are the other Spleen relationships? In the previous chapters.

SPLEEN AND KIDNEY

This is a relationship of Body Fluids and Qi.

Spleen (Earth)	Kidney (Water)
Root of Post-heaven/postnatal Qi • Produces Qi and Blood from food and drink intake.	Root of Pre-heaven/prenatal Qi • Holds/stores Yuan Qi and acquired Essence, which supplements congenital Essence
Middle source (MJ) of water • Produces water that is sent to LU and KI	Lower source (LJ) of water • Controls water/fluid metabolism

Many overweight patients are in the condition they are in because of a Spleen and Kidney Deficiency. Water metabolism then accumulates in the abdomen and lower extremities. This can be exacerbated by a Kidney Yang Deficiency, which has symptoms of cold and often diarrhea in the early morning (5am), especially cold in the lower extremities and in the waist.

This page intentionally left blank

CHAPTER 9
Yang Inter-relationships

There are four Yang organ interrelationships to know. And I mean memorize the stuff next to the numbers that I bolded. The stuff underneath is just a little explanation to help you remember.

1. **Most Yang organs are *anatomically connected.***
    The Yin relationships are connected by their channel relationships, but the yang organs have an anatomical association. The Urinary Bladder (BL), for instance, is connected through the San Jiao.

2. **Qi descends in all six Yang organs.**

3. **All Yang organs involve digestion and excretion.**

4. **All Yang organs have Stomach as their center.**
    Therefore, if you adjust the Stomach organ, you basically affect all other Yang organs.

There are also some Yin/Yang organ relationships, but you already know about these because they are the paired organ relationships: Spleen/Stomach, Lung/Large Intestine, Heart/Small Intestine, Kidney/Bladder, Liver/Gallbladder.

These are based on *channel distribution*, not anatomical relationship! As one example, the Heart channel runs on the medial side of the arm and is considered the more internal channel compared to its' paired organ, the Small Intestine. The Small Intestine channel is more lateral and exterior, even running on the lateral side of the arm.

This page intentionally left blank

SECTION 3: CHANNELS AND COLLATERALS

This is the world's shortest section, but deserves some specific press.

Channels or meridians are the main "highways" of energy/Qi. They carry Qi, nutrients, and more good stuff around the body. Collaterals (also called connecting channels) are like smaller roads branching off the main 'highway.'

It is important to know how each of these connect and where they go so that you understand the whole picture. I think it's also worth noting that there is a branch of Chinese medicine that treats pain and other things primarily based on the channels and collaterals. There's an excellent book called *Applied Channel Theory in Chinese Medicine: Wang Ju-Yi's Lectures on Channel Therapeutics*. Super awesome. Check it out in your local school library someday after you've finished all of your Foundations studies, Point Locations and Energetics, and Diagnostics. But don't check it out *this* day. It'll just get confusing.

This page intentionally left blank

CHAPTER 10
Channels and Collaterals

Once you start reading Chinese medical literature, checking stuff our in your school library and such, you will find multiple terms for just about any concept in Chinese medicine. The main channels/meridians and collaterals/connecting channels are no exception. Channels are often called meridians in literature you will read. I'll use both terms just to help your mind flex a little. ☺

There are twelve *regular meridians*, all of which have acupuncture points along them. Each of the six Zang and six Fu organ (as you can see in the following table) has an associated meridian, giving you the twelve regular meridians.

There are also eight *extraordinary meridians*. Most of them don't have points, but two of them do (the Ren and Du channels), so they are sometimes grouped in with the Regular Meridians. Just be aware that the Ren and Du channel can shift back and forth in the groupings, but for the purpose of tests, keep those Ren and Du channels in the extraordinary set. You can use acupuncture points to affect the extraordinary channels, but you have to "borrow" combinations of them from the channels that have points in order to work with them.

Meridian/channel breakdown

Meridian name	Channel Category	Does it have points?
Lung	Regular meridian/channel	Yes
Large Intestine		
Stomach		
Spleen		
Heart		
Small Intestine		
Urinary Bladder		
Kidney		
Pericardium		
San Jiao		
Gallbladder		
Liver		
Ren/Conception Vessel	Extraordinary channel/vessel	
Du/Governing Vessel		
Chong/Penetrating Vessel		No
Dai/Girdling or Belt Vessel		
Yin Qiao or Yin Motility		
Yang Qiao or Yang Motility		
Yin Wei or Yin Linking		
Yang Wei or Yang Linking		

Fun thing to know about the extraordinary vessels: Jerry Alan Johnson says in his book, *Chinese Medical Qigong Therapy, Vol. 1: Energetic Anatomy and Physiology* that the extraordinary vessels are the first ones formed in the body in utero and the other channels are layered around it as we develop. That means they are very deep in the body, not on the surface, hence the lack of acupuncture points.

Besides the regular and extraordinary channels, there are also the following, each flowing from their associated *regular* channel:
- 12 tendino-muscular channels
- 12 divergent channels
- 12 skin or cutaneous channels

There are also 15 collateral channels (also called connecting or Luo channels), one from each of the 12 regular meridians and one each from the Du and Ren channels. If you add that up, you only get 14 channels. Where is the 15th? The Spleen has an extra one called The Great Luo of the Spleen.

If you're doing the math, adding all of these up, that's seventy one channels and collaterals. My professor, Dr. Wu, said there is also one more connecting the Spleen/Stomach to the Heart, making 72. If you've already had a Points/Energetics class or two, these will sound familiar. If you haven't, that can sound very overwhelming. Be patient with yourself. Trust you're going to get it. You don't memorize all of this at once, just little bits at a time, adding to your overall knowledge. Hang in there!

FUNCTIONS OF THE CHANNELS AND COLLATERALS

There are five to know. This isn't tested that much from what I've seen, but you'd do well to understand it nonetheless.

Function	Explanation
Connects the body together as an energetic whole	Like an energetic infrastructure. It's not a part of it at all, but it is similar to the nervous system in that it links everything together. • Connects the internal organs and five sense organs. • Connects the internal organs to the extremities, which is why you can needle the acupuncture points on the surface and it has an effect on the organs. • Connects the internal organs with the soft tissues

Pathway for Qi and Blood	While the blood vessels, as understood in biomedicine, are not the same thing as the meridians, it is nonetheless proper to say that the blood vessel system is *part* of the channel system, due to the Blood pathway connection.
Conducts sensations	I'm not talking nerve sensations of pain, heat, cold, etc. That's a biomed thing. This refers to the broader definition of Shen, which is carried via Wei Qi and Ying Qi. The movement of Wei, Ying, and Yuan Qi that is stimulated by acupuncture manipulation can be *felt* by both the practitioner and the patient. That's the kind of sensation I mean. And that sensation is experienced differently by every individual.
Pathways of Evil Qi	This is related to the channels and collaterals being a pathway for Qi and Blood. Pathogens and pathogenic influences take opportunistic advantage of this same pathway system in much the same way that an invading army captures roads, bridges, and supply lines. FYI, "evil" doesn't mean truly evil, just refers to its' effect on the body. Evil in that it causes dis-ease and disharmony.
Helps to regulate excess and deficiency, Yin and Yang	Qi and Blood, Yin and Yang are transferred around the body as needed using these pathways. If there is an area that is deficient, you can use acupuncture to help the resources move around where they need to be.

APPLICATION OF CHANNEL/COLLATERAL THEORY

You can use channel and collateral theory to good effect in Chinese medicine in four areas: physiology, pathology, diagnosis, and treatment.

Physiology

In physiology, channel and collateral theory explains the interrelation of the organs we discussed in the previous section. Through the channels and collaterals all of the parts of the body are connected together in an organic whole.

In Pathology

Pathogens travel from one organ to another. The six evils go from the superficial to the internal organs in this order:

> Skin/cutaneous channels on the surface of the body → tendino-muscular channels → collateral channels → divergent channels → regular meridians → extraordinary meridians at the deepest level of the body.

If you have an ill patient, do not open the confluent points, which are a direct pathway to the deepest part of the body! Example: Spleen 4 on the foot is a confluent point for the Chong Meridian.

Some practitioners also feel that you should stick with (pardon the pun) the upper body points when a person comes in with an illness that is still on the exterior part of the body so that it is not drawn deeper down into the body.

In Diagnosis

Points along the channel pathway of an organ that has a problem of some kind are often tender. As an example, if a patient has pneumonia, the LU 1 and LU 2 points on the chest near the shoulder will be tender and BL 13 on the upper back will too. LU 1 and LU 2 are on the Lung channel and BL 13 is Back Shu point of the Lung – an influential point or Lung problems.

In biomedicine, one of the diagnostic tests for fibromyalgia is palpation on 18 different points that are known to be reactive. Most of these are acupuncture points. If the patient has tenderness at 9 or more of these points, this is considered an indicator of fibromyalgia.

In Treatment

Herbs work first on the channels and secondarily on the organs. All herbs have actions on the channels, which you will eventually memorize in Intro to Herbs and the regular single herb classes. Some guide to channels as well. You can add guide to channel herbs to usher the other herbs to where you want them to go.

Additionally, sometimes dysfunction isn't a problem of the *organ* but of the channel, which is blocked or stagnant or deficient in some way. Acupuncture, herbs, and medical Qigong can open these channels and restore them to proper function.

I remember being blown away when I was in student clinic by a licensed practitioner I interned with who treated from a channel perspective. A guy came in complaining of sciatica along the right lateral leg, pain in the right side of his neck, and tight spot on his forehead just above the right eyebrow. The practitioner asked a few questions and pointed out to me that all of the painful spots were along the Gallbladder channel. After doing some palpation for tenderness along a couple of channels, he inserted only four points based on his knowledge of channel theory, *none of which* were on the Gallbladder channel by the way, and the guys tightness and pain were completely released within 30 minutes. Yeah. Clinic fun!

SECTION 4: FOUNDATION OF DIAGNOSTICS

By the time you get to this section, you know about Yin and Yang, Five Element Theory, Zangfu Theory, and you've studied the bejesus out of the organ systems and channel systems. Now we are moving on to etiology, pathogenic influences (internal, external, and emotional in nature), mechanisms of disease, diagnosis, and treatment.

You'll get *way* more of this in diagnostic studies, in point location, in energetics and more. This is just laying the groundwork for that. Grasp the 101-ness of this and you will make your life easier later!

This page intentionally left blank

CHAPTER 11
Etiology

In a Western medical definition, etiology refers to the cause or causes of disease.

More importantly for us at the momet, from a Chinese medical perspective, *etiology refers to the pathogenic factors causing Yin/Yang disorder (or disharmony) and the internal organ problems resulting in sickness.*

CHARACTERISTICS OF CHINESE MEDICINE ETIOLOGIES

There are three characteristics of a Chinese Etiology:

Characteristics	Explanation
"Cause of disease" is a relative term	Cause of disease = pathogenic factors. Why is this relative? Because pathogenic factors don't affect every person the same. Think about allergies – cedar pollen may affect this person, but not that one. For the person affected, this is a pathogenic factor. For the person who is not, this is not a pathogen!
Pathogenic factors have their susceptibility	Specific pathogens tend to attack specific organs. Examples <ul><li>Wind affects Liver strongly</li><li>Anger also strongly affects the Liver</li><li>Cold affects the Lungs</li><li>Damp affects the Spleen</li><li>Fear negatively impacts the Kidney</li></ul>
Pathogenic factors are closely related to symptomatology	Biomedicine relies on technical testing to find pathogens while we don't. Diagnosis in Chinese medicine is based on sets of s/sx. This exterior forensic method indicates the balance of both Yin and Yang as well as of the Zangfu.

CATEGORIES OF ETIOLOGY IN CHINESE MEDICINE

There are also three categories of etiology in Chinese medicine.

Etiology category	Brief discussion
External pathogens	These are the six evils: Wind, Cold, Heat, Summer Heat, Dry, and Damp. Summer heat is heat + damp and only affects the body during the summer season – like literally June 21-Sept 21. For real. In many cases there is a kind of "incubation" period for external evils. Like a wind invasion has a period of a few hours to a day or so from invasion to signs and symptoms.
Internal pathogens	This refers to the seven emotional disorders. No incubation period for this! It's pretty instantaneous. These seven emotions are linked to the internal Yin organs.
Non-internal, non-external pathogens	This is stuff like poor diet, overwork, insect bites, accidents, sports injuries, inadequate or too much sleep, etc. It can even include environmental toxins, exposure to too much bright light or sound, etc.

PATHOGENS AT DIFFERENT LIFE PERIODS

Different periods in life open you up to different pathogenic influences.

Life period	Brief discussion and notes
Prenatal period	Any substance which passes from the mother to the child during pregnancy or during labor and delivery can be a prenatal pathogen. The *quantity* and *quality* of Essence, especially Preheaven Essence, sets the tone for a person's life-long constitution. This applies not only to genetic/inherited disease, but also to the development of hypertension, diabetes, high cholesterol, etc. These, along with genetic dysfunction or damage, are all the result of poor

	congenital essence passed from the parents to the child. Did you ever wonder why some people get cancer while other people with the same diet, lifestyle, and exposure don't? This is one reason why. Fetal toxins are poisons from the mother and can include chemicals and drugs. During breast feeding the mother can help counter this by taking tiny amounts of da huang. This herb is good for clearing fetal toxins and toxic heat. This will keep the child from having problems of constipation or skin later on. Abortions or miscarriages reduce the Qi in the mother. Wait 3-5 months afterwards before attempting conception again. The mother should have regular periods at least 3 times to ensure the Kidney Qi has been restored sufficiently to support a fetus. Consider the season: Autumn is the best time to conceive a child as the parental essence is stored at this time, banked up if you will. Shock or upset or divorce during pregnancy, difficult labor or forceps delivery all increase the chance of epilepsy and emotional/mental problems.
Childhood period	There are three major types of pathogens that tend to affect kids in this period. Childrens' internal organs are still fragile and developing during this period and they don't handle this level of pathogens well. • The Six Evils These are the biggies during childhood and include cross contamination from other little kids – like when colds and flus sweep through daycare centers or when a family just keeps passing the same stomach bug between them. • Irregular Diet Cokes, candy, sweets, cheese, snacks, and a lack of fresh vegetables all = irregular diet. • Emotional Disorders Abusive parents, unstable home, a parent with an anger problem, etc. These will affect kids long term. As an example, abused kids often grow up to have adult-onset asthma, joint pain, and more. This

	is tied to the emotional environment in which this (former) child developed.
Adult period	"Adult" is calculated differently for females and males: women become adults at 21 (because they have 7 year cycles in life) while men are considered adults at 24 (8 year cycles).
	The predominant pathogen adults is that of lifestyle. Lifestyle generates emotional and stress reactions. Diseases that grow from this source include hypertension, high blood sugar, high cholesterol.

CHAPTER 12
Pathogenic Influences: Emotional Disorders

Emotions are normal for humans. They only become pathogenic when one or more of them causes problems. This generally happens when emotions become "toxic."

I've heard more than one spiritual teacher say this: emotions are normal when you experience them, then they flow away. If they last more than 20 minutes or so, they have become toxic and will affect your health.

THE SEVEN EMOTIONS

The seven basic emotions are:
- Joy
- Anger
- Fear
- Grief
- Worry
- Pensiveness (thinking about stuff)
- Shock

In and of themselves, there is nothing wrong with these emotions. So when do they become abnormal or pathogenic? This happens in three ways. All of these interfere with one's life and cause sickness. . . or lack of health.

When emotions attack....	Brief discussion
Suddenness of onset	When a strong emotion hits you and you had no warning it was coming, this can become a pathological influence. One example might be the sudden death of a loved one. Or the 911 attacks.

Strength of the emotion	Overwhelming emotion, for instance. This refers to the amount of emotion released at once.
Chronic in nature	Maybe not as violent as the one above, but repeats over and over again. Kind of an emotional repetitive strain problem. Similar to how chronic stress is linked to chronic systemic inflammation.

Dis-ease due to pathological emotional influence has three common characteristics.

Characteristic of pathological emotions	Brief discussion
No incubation period	Attack the internal organs directly and suddenly. The *Neijing* says the emotions derive from the five organs. When they are out of balance, they can then become *internal* pathogens. Here are a couple of examples. An abnormal and constant state of anger can negatively impact the Liver. Postpartum depression can lead to Liver Qi and Blood deficiencies . . . and Liver Qi and Blood problems can lead to postpartum depression in much the same way that PMS is both the cause and aggravator of Liver Qi stagnation.*
They affect transportation of Qi	Normal Qi movements are affected by the emotions. Anger, for instance causes Qi to ascend. Fear causes it to descend. Worry and overthinking cause Qi to stagnate.
Chronic emotional disorder causes heat and fire	That's because a chronic state of emotional disorder leads to stagnation. Stagnation leads to heat and fire. **

*Not only can the emotions cause organ disharmony, emotions can likewise follow based on the condition of the internal organs. Just another fun benefit of the inter-relation between the energy world and the physical world

**It took me a while to wrap my brain around this one. Think about water. A running stream is always cooler than a swampy non-moving body of water. If it rains hard for instance, the stream of runoff is cool in temperature. But if it pools in a flat spot in your yard and sits there it gets hot and swampy. This happens in the body too. Anywhere there is no circulation there is stagnancy and heat.

DISORDERS OF THE SEVEN EMOTIONS

OK, let's break down the seven emotions and see what this looks like when you're face to face with it in clinic.

Anger

Anger makes Qi rise and strongly affects the Liver. When Qi ascends too much, this is Qi rebellion and can result in Liver Qi Rebellion syndrome. This is what that looks like:

Anger s/sx	Brief discussion
Throbbing headache	This is too much Qi rising and getting "stuck" at the head. Like a balloon bumping against the ceiling, but more pissed off.
Dizziness and/or vertigo	Both Qi rising up and Wind associated with the element of Wood/Liver.
Irritability	Points to the chronic nature of this anger – always lurking around, always close to the surface. Also about the heat that this kind of syndrome produces. Internal heat frequently = irritability.
Elevated blood pressure	Not necessarily a medical diagnosis of hypertension, but anger and stress do constrict the blood vessels and cause an elevated pressure.
Red eyes and face	Heat generated by the anger affecting the complexion of the face. Heat rises with the Qi.
Shaking, tremors of extremities	This also has to do with the Wood element associated with Liver and how Wind affects it. Anger makes the Qi ascend, causes some heat and those together generate an internal Wind.
Pulse: wiry Tongue: could be normal	Wiry pulse is frequently associated with Liver disharmony.

Treat Liver Qi Rebellion Syndrome with an acupuncture pattern called The Four Gates: LV 3 + LI 4. Add Du 20 at the top of the head.

From a Five Element perspective, there is an old practice of treating one emotion with another. Grief or sadness (associated with Metal), for instance, will control the anger (associated with the wood element). This reminds me of some old 1950's movies I've seen. When someone is hysterical in those movies (Liver and Heart) another character slaps the raving person (shock – scatters the rising Qi) and they calm down. Seems a little harsh to me, but this wisdom has been around a lot longer than I have, so who ya gonna listen to?

Joy

The *Neijing* says that when Ying Qi and Wei qi flow smoothly, there is happiness. Well, what about too much happiness, too much joy? What the heck is wrong with being joyful? Nada. But for there to be health, there must be balance.

Too much joy is referred to as "overjoy" in the old manuscript translations. Overjoy from a western perspective could be called *mania*. Overjoy causes the Qi flow to slow down an affects the Heart. This excess of joy scatters the Heart Qi and as a result scatters the Shen too.

Have you ever laughed at something so much that you couldn't inhale from the laughter? If you keep on, eventually your limbs start to feel a little weak, you can't catch your breath, your eyes tear, and you start slapping things – your thighs, your chest. Your body is doing that automatically to manually move the Qi.

Let's look at symptoms of "Overjoy" or Mania. And these aren't from laughing too much at a joke. This is more of a toxic problem. As a matter of fact, my dad had a serious heart attack around 2001 and his symptoms looked a lot like this.

Overjoy s/sx	Brief discussion
Shortness of breath	Qi slows down and scatters, affects the Heart. Heart Qi and Shen are also scattered.
Chest tightness or stuffiness	
Palpitation	
Pale face turning to purple	Due to lack of blood flow, condition of Heart showing on face
Pulse: intermittent or moderate (55-60bpm) *or* slow and uneven pulse.	

From a Five Element perspective, treat overjoy with fear. My professor told a story about a man who had been trying to pass a civil service exam for many tries. When he finally passed he celebrated and got pretty manic. So his family told him his wife was in grave danger (which wasn't true). This fear snapped him out of his reverie and he broke the "spell" or cycle of the condition of overjoy. Again, seems a bit harsh? IDK.

Worry and Pensiveness

Doesn't matter if you call it worry, pensiveness, overthinking, or ruminating thoughts. Either way, an obsessive internal dialogue is occurring over and over again. And all of them same basic effect: they slow the movement of Qi and can strongly impact the Spleen. The emotional disorders referred to as colitis, gastritis of the stomach or duodenum, or IBS can all have their root in Spleen dysfunction and could arise from worry and pensiveness.

Worry/Pensiveness s/sx	Brief discussion
Appetite: decreased, poor or none.	Qi is not moving downward or isn't moving quickly enough. Food movement is sluggish which is an excess of food, so the body doesn't want more.
Abdominal fullness	Qi isn't moving through the area, so it feels full.
Abdominal distention	Belly might look distended and could feel hard.

Gas and bloating	Qi isn't moving, so stuff builds up that is usually released.
Loose stool with undigested food or diarrhea	Spleen can't process the food you eat, so food is passed through the intestines instead of being processed.
Tongue:	Pale, swollen tongue body with possible teethmarks. White coating.
Pulse: Wiry	Wiry? Wiry is usually associated with the Liver, but not always.

Sadness and Grief

Aren't sadness and grief normal, especially after a loss? Yes, they are. So is re-experiencing a sense of loss, sadness, and/or grief on the anniversaries of that loss. But when it persists for years without a break it becomes an abnormal situation.

Sadness and grief dissolve Qi and strongly affect the Lung. Sadness and grief can cause the Heart to become cramped and agitated, which is then pushed to the lobes of the Lungs. Wei Qi and Yin become blocked. This creates heat and fire, which dissolves Qi.

Sadness and Grief s/sx	Brief discussion
Shortness of breath	Weakness of the Lung Qi
Soft, weak voice	
Diminished immunity	Lung cannot feed the Wei Qi, so immunity suffers
Catches cold easily	
Chest tightness and stagnation	Qi cannot move in the chest, so there is stagnation in the chest. Sighing is also a Liver Qi stagnation sign, but that's because Liver cannot circulate Qi through the chest. This is occurring because Lung Qi cannot circulate in the chest due to the dissolution of Qi.
Sighing from time to time	

Treat the Lung by tonifying Lung Qi. Untreated, allergies and shortness of breath can occur among other symptoms you will learn in your Diagnostics studies. Symptoms will improve when Lung Qi is improved.

Fear

In the classic tradition, fear and shock were grouped together. Recent thought in Chinese medicine separates them, probably due to advanced in the study of psychology. Note that shock is an acute reaction to an external stimulus while fear is a more chronic pattern and is more internal.

Fear causes the Qi to descend and negatively impacts the Kidneys. Some people totally lose control of their bladder when they are very afraid. This is Qi descending due to fear and Kidney losing the ability to control the lower two openings. Over time, fear can cause Kidney Qi prolapse symptoms.

Long term fear s/sx	Brief discussion
Frequent urination, incontinence	Kidney can no longer control the lower two openings
Miscarriage	A happy womb and proper fetal development rely heavily on the Kidneys. Kidneys weakened by fear have a more difficult time supporting a developing baby.
Fullness and a sinking feeling in the lower abdomen	Qi cannot move in the lower abdomen and begins to feel full. The sinking feeling is tied to the conditions ripe for prolapse.
Fatigue	Kidney Qi helps you have energy to get life done. Fear causes the Qi to descend and leave less "umph" for life.
Pulse: Deep	Reflects the deeply internal aspect of the dysfunction.

Shock

Shock is an acute reaction to an external stimulus. Shock scatters the Qi and affects the Heart and Kidney. It first affects the Heart and then the Shen. The Kidney becomes involved and Qi scatters.

Shock s/sx	Brief discussion
Acute panic attack	Heart involvement. Fear of dying, loss of control, fatigue, exhaustion
Incontinence of urine or stool	This is the Kidney involvement – cannot control the two lower openings.
Pulse: Indistinctive	Difficult to feel, not clear.

Chapter 13
Pathogenic Influences: The Six Evils

Liu Yin is the Pinyin version of the Chinese term that means "six evils." And no, it's not the same Yin as in Yin and Yang. Different accent and intonation, different character in Chinese.

In an of themselves, these "evils" simply aren't evil. They derive from the Liu Qi – the Six Qi. They only become "evil" when they become excessive and/or enter the body and cause disharmony leading to disease. The Six Qi come from your natural environment.

The Six Qi	
Wind	Summer Heat*
Cold	Heat or Fire
Damp	Dryness

*Summer heat is damp + heat and is specific to the summer season.

Weather causes changes in pressure, temperature, and humidity. Pressure changes lead to the formation of wind. Temperature changes bring cold or heat. Humidity is responsible for conditions of dryness (lack of humidity) and dampness.

Summer heat is both a season and a climate change. Summer heat is a combination of damp and heat. By definition, it can only occur between Summer Solstice and the Autumnal Equinox! The *Neijing* says if you suffer from Yang, heat, and/or fire prior to or after the Summer Solstice, you have a Heat or Fire Invasion.

WHEN THE SIX QI BECOME THE SIX EVILS

Liu Qi (Six Qi) becomes the Six Evils under the conditions noted in the table below. Remember that if it doesn't make you sick, then it's not an evil! These things are all relative, not absolute!

When the Six Qi "attack:"
1. When one of the Six Qi is too strong, abnormally strong, or excessive
2. When the Six Qi occur out of season
3. When the weather changes too quickly
4. When one or all of the above is true in addition to a deficiency or drop in the body's ability to defend from it.

General characteristics of an invasion of the Six Evils

There are four of these to know.

Characteristic	Brief discussion
Invasion of the 6 Evils relates to weather, climate change and seasonal changes as well as to the geographic conditions, external environmental factors, and living/working conditions.	In Spring, for example, it is common to experience Wind Invasion. In Autumn, one is more prone to Dryness. In Summer people tend to get dermatitis due to sweat pores being blocked. Regarding geographical conditions, the *NeiJing* says that people who life in the East experience more wind invasions. (Remember that this was written for a Chinese audience man years ago – the East in China is on the coast, which is much windier. People in the west side of china live in dryness, while people in the south are subject to heat and fire invasions. Different areas in China have different treatment principles due to the variation in climate, which is how different schools of treatment philosophies and practices arose. For instance, the *Shang Han Lun* is all about Cold diseases. Another treatise in Chinese Medicine is the Wen Bin Xue, the *Treatise on Warm Diseases*. For a more local example, if you lived in Seattle you'd be treating far more damp and cold than you would in Phoenix or Austin where you're more likely to treat wind and heat.

When the Six Evils invade the body, it's usually multiple pathogens that invade.	Wind is the primary one, but it's far less common to have just a wind invasion than it is to have a wind cold, wind heat, wind damp heat, etc type invasion. Wind opens the door of the body more easily than most of the Six Qi and brings friends along for the ride. Arthritis, for example, is generally wind cold or wind damp invasions. A cold with copious sticky mucus might be wind damp cold or wind damp heat.
After the Six Evils invade, the property of the Six Evils can be changed	Cold can convert to heat or fire or dry for instance. When someone gets a cold invasion, for instance, s/sx include nasal drainage, fatigue, a light fever and body aches, the tongue will have a thin whie coating, all indicative of a cold invasion. Within 2-5 days there is yellow discharge, darker urine, constipation, higher fever. These signs indicate heat. A body's constitution decides how, when, and if the changes occur. A "fire" person who gets an invasion of damp will manifest a damp heat. A water person who gets a cold invasion manifests a damp cold. It also depends upon what you consume -- when you eat fiery foods you introduce fire into the body, when you eat damp foods you introduce damp into the body. If you have a cold invasion and eat damp foods, you can get damp/cold. Another factor is how long you have an invasion. If it stays around long enough it will convert to heat and fire.
The Six Evils invade the body through the skin (sweating pores), the five sense organs, and the two lower orifices	The sense organs are natural openings from the organs to the external environment. The openings that are invaded are the ones affected. For example, if the nose is invaded you get an itchy nose, if the eyes are invaded they will be watery or dry and itchy. The site of attack, in other words, is the one affected. Wind, cold and dry evils of a Yin nature while damp, heat and summer heat are Yang evils.

This is a breakdown of each of the Six Evils and how they affect the body.

Wind Evil

Wind can affect the body at any time, but is most predominant in the Spring season. The places that are most susceptible to invasion are:

Common site of invasion	Brief discussion
Skin and sweating pores	The Wei Qi level – and thus the Lung is involved.
Sense organs	These orifices into the body are susceptible to the invasion of wind.
Wind points	Gb 20, Sj 17, Du 16, Si 12, Bl 12, and Gb 31 Most of these points are on the head, back of the neck and upper back. Gb 31 on the lateral thigh is a lower body wind point.

Pathogenic characteristics

If you can understand the pathogenic characteristics of wind it will help you in clinic quite a lot. There are five characteristics of a wind invasion that you need to understand.

Characteristic	Brief discussion
Wind is a Yang pathogen and tends to attack the Yang areas.	Yang areas are above the waist, mostly on the head, face and the five sense organs. This is where all of the Yang meridians meet. The skin, superficial areas, and back are also Yang in nature. The Du channel, which runs up the spine is considered to be the Sea of Yang. Generally speaking, if the location of a symptom is in a Yang area, then Wind is involved.

A wind evil tends to case sweating.	Generally speaking, a patient that catches a cold and sweats has a wind invasion. A patient that catches a cold and doesn't sweat has a cold invasion. Wind opens the sweating pores and holds them open. Cold closes them tightly.
Wind evils change quickly and move quickly.	Any wind invasion must be of acute onset. It causes wandering symptoms. Environmentally, wind works in this way too. If symptoms move around then it's probably wind causing it.
Wind evil is a guide for other pathogens.	Wind is often accompanied by and is a carrier for other evils such as cold, heat or damp. Wind is dynamic and pervasive. Other pathogens then follow the Wind and invade the body. Qi and Body Fluids become weak with a wind invasion and are then more susceptible to other pathogens.
Wind causes an itching sensation.	Allergies and hives are a classic example of this.

Manifestations of Wind

All types of allergies are wind invasions, including food allergies. Common cold is another as are arthritis and Bell's Palsy.

Symptoms of Wind

Don't confuse internal and external wind. Exterior wind looks like this:

Wind s/sx	Brief discussion
Acute onset	S/sx show up suddenly. External wind is never chronic.
Location of s/sx on upper body	Head, five sense organs, face, neck, and upper back

This includes respiratory and sense organ affected allergies. Even allergies such as allergies to pet dander, dust mites, and newsprint inks still come down to wind.

Interiorly generated wind is longer term with a slower onset. Interior wind often comes with twitches and tremors.

Best way to treat wind? Acupuncture.

Cold Evil

Cold is predominant in the winter. Kind of a duh, I know. If you travel below the equator, however, the script is flipped and cold becomes predominant in a whole different season.

Pathogenic Characteristics

Three characteristics you need to understand.

Characteristics	Brief discussion
Cold is a Yin pathogen and tends to attack and injure Yang, making Yang weak and deficient.	If you look at the six stages for cold injured diseases (diseases caused by cold invasion) in the *Shang Han Lun* you see that the Yang is slowly worn down. The herbs in the *Shang Han Lun* are geared toward preserving and saving Yang. The Six Stages are: Taiyang, Yang Ming, ShaoYang, Tai Yin, Shao Yin, Jue Yin. As one is exhausted, the evil moves to the next one. Yang becomes less and less in each stage as the cold attacks it. Yang is the defending energy in this case. If you save Yang, you can stop the development of the disease.

Cold causes blockage and coagulation.	Think of an iced up river. The coagulation of the Blood, Body Fluids, and Essence causes swelling, edema, joint pain, headaches, and arthritis. Menstruation, when affected by cold yields cramping and pain. This blockage and coagulation produces the symptoms of cold, body and joint pains, headaches, stiff neck, pale face turning to blue/purple and blue/purple/pale nails, overall stiffness.
Cold contracts the body tissues and closes off the sweat pores, so you get goose bumps, but no sweating.	Cold produces the symptoms of spasms, stiffness, all types of headaches, body aches, and a lack of sweating (because cold closes off the sweating pores).

Signs and Symptoms of a Cold Invasion

Cold Evil Invasion s/sx – no discussion	
Chills	No sweating
Aversion to cold	Pale face, becoming purple over time
Pain (#1 sx seen in clinic for cold invasion)	Pale nails or bluish purple nails
Stiffness overall	Cold extremities
Stiffness in neck	Cough with watery or white loose mucus
Body and joint pains	Spasms
Headaches of all types	Pulse: superficial, tight

Common diseases of cold invasion include common cold, headaches, and arthritis. The Lung is especially susceptible to wind and cold invasions.

Damp Evil

The most common season for a damp evil is what is called Long Summer in China. This describes a season at the end of summer and just before autumn arrives when damp is more prevalent. There are 5 seasons in China: spring, summer, long summer, autumn and winter. This fits into the Five Element model. This condition accelerates the communication between heaven and earth. At this time summer heat will often invade the body accompanied by dampness.

The most common organ to be attacked by a dampness evil is the Spleen. Spleen controls digestion, transforming food and water and extracting the prana, Qi or essence from them. Dampness causes digestion problems such as poor appetite, loose stool and nausea.

Think of dampness as stickiness – like when it's really humid outside, enough so that your clothes stick to your skin. That kind of humidity makes it hard to move around and saps the energy. I also think of damp in the Spleen like a kind of sticky mud that you try to walk through and it sucks the shoes off of your feet. Definitely hard to make any headway walking through the muck

Pathogenic Characteristics

There are four major characteristics and some minor sub-characteristics you need to understand about damp.

Characteristics	Brief discussion
Damp evil tends to attack the lower parts of the body.	Specifically, the 2 lower orifices. A UTI (urinary tract infection) is a good example of this. If a person goes to the doc with s/sx of a UTI the will be tested for bacteria in the urine. Bacteria can be either gram positive (G+) or gram negative (G-). Gram positive bacteria attack the upper body, so it is a Yang pathogen (skin infections, throat infections, mastitis, dermatitis,

	carbuncles, etc). Gram negative bacteria on the other hand cause UTI. Gram negative bacteria are Yin pathogens. Any pathogen transmited via Body Fluids is considered to be a Yin pathogen, including STDs.
Damp evil is turbid and heavy.	Comes with both of these symptoms. Turbidity = • Turbid excretions – BM is sticky and stinky, vaginal discharge is thick and sticky, urine is cloudy, eye discharge is thick Heaviness = • Heavy tight head, heaviness in limbs. Heaviness is always damp associated. Also associated with dampness = • Foggy thinking, unclear thinking, confusion, sleepy sensations during the day.
Dampness is sticky	• Excretions are sticky • Tongue has sticky, slippery or greasy coating • Makes other diseases and syndromes harder to get rid of because dampness acts like a kind of glue for this.
Dampness is a Yin evil: it tends to block Qi and damage Yang.	Blocks Spleen and Stomach Qi so that Spleen Qi cannot rise and Stomach Qi cannot descend, causing s/sx like diarrhea, gas, bloating, nausea and vomiting, low or no appetite. This sounds a lot like Stomach flu, HIV, hepatitis, yes? That's because all viral infections are dampness, either damp + heat or damp + cold. Virals are transmitted through fluids, which makes them a Yin pathogen.

	When the Spleen gets blocked it generally results in damage of the Spleen Yang, so even if you didn't start with a cold condition, this will generate one. And cold + damp damages Yang further, causing more Yang deficiency rather directly. Ain't that a fun game?

Signs and Symptoms of a Damp Invasion

Look at all that damp, sticky, turbid stuff going on in this list.

S/Sx of a Damp Invasion	Brief elaboration
Turbidity of excretions	See above
Stickiness of excretions	Urine, stools, eye, vaginal discharge, and nasal discharge will be thick and sticky.
Viral infections	Damp and Yin in nature
Heavy sensations	Heaviness of the head, with or without a tight band feeling around the head. Heavy sensations in the limbs.
Foggy sensations	Foggy head, foggy mind, unclear thinking, confusion, sleepy sensations during the day (not associated with bedtime).
Spleen and Stomach Qi problems	Like diarrhea, gas, bloating, nausea, vomiting, poor or no appetite.
Tongue coatings will be sticky, slippery, or greasy looking	Reflecting the nature of the dampness.
Pulse will be slippery	When you feel the pulse you use your index, middle and ring finger and you feel a slippery pulse, it feels like beads moving under each finger one at a time. The sensation reminds me of how it feels when you drum your fingers on the table,

	except you aren't the one doing the drumming—the pulse is.

Summer Heat Evil

Neijing says that summer heat is very much related to the change of the seasons. As a matter of fact, it's the only evil closely related to seasonal changes. It's also the only pathogen that can only come in from outside – other pathogens can arise internally because they can be indigenous in the body, but not this one. You can only get an invasion of summer heat between the Summer Solstice (June 20 or 21) and the Autumnal Equinox (Sept 22 or 23).

Pathogenic Characteristics

There are four major characteristics and some minor subcharacteristics you need to understand about summer heat evils.

Characteristics	Brief discussion
Summer heat is a Yang pathogen that causes Yang s/sx.	Red face, fever, sweating, constipation, thirst, desire for cold drinks, urine that is dark yellow, hot and burning. Pulse will be fast and forceful while the tongue will be red in the body and yellow in the coating. When you look at the Four Greats (big fever, big pulse, big thirst, big sweating) you see them in the s/sx above.
Summer heat evil consumes Qi and Body Fluids. • Causes Qi deficiency • Causes dehydration	Because it causes Qi deficiency, it also damages Body Fluids. Dehydration is Body Fluid deficiency. Body Fluids carry the Qi, so when they are deficient so is Qi.

Summer heat often invades with body in combination with dampness.	A high fever, sweating, red face plus loose stool, diarrhea, heaviness, nausea/vomiting and low or no appetite is summer heat + damp
Summer heat evil tends to attack the Heart and Pericardium.	Heart and Pericardium fire elements. Summer heat immediately attacks the Blood and the Heart. The result is insomnia, irritability, tossing and turning, tachycardia.

There are three very handy herbs to use for Summer Heat Invasions. hua shi (talc), he ye (lotus leaf), and xi gua cui yi (green watermelon rind. Three hand foods to combat summer heat: mung beans, mung bean sprouts, and winter melon (from an oriental grocery store). You can get mung beans and sprouts at Whole Foods. If you can't find the sprouts, they are deadly easy to sprout in your kitchen cabinet. You need a paper towel, a water sprayer/mister, and mung beans. Look it up. Super simple, and really tasty stuff.

Dryness Evil

Dryness is predominant in autumn. Autumn is Yin. The coolness of autumn slows communication between heaven and earth so the humidity drops and a condition of dryness occurs. As the Yin and Yang properties of a dryness evil are unclear, there are many debates in the Chinese medicine community as to whether dryness is one or the other. Hmmm. Autumn is definitely a Yin season, yet dry is more Yang in nature while Yin is wet. At the onset of the season it's still warm which suggests Yang. But at the end of autumn it's cold and dry which is more Yin in nature. Hmmm again

Pathogenic Characteristics

There are only two to know this time with some elaboration.

Characteristics	Brief discussion
Dryness is astringent and causes dry s/sx.	Astringency blocks and contracts. The s/sx are all dry: dry skin, hair, mouth, lips, nose, scanty urine, etc. More on that below. Astringency also suppresses the Lung Qi's dispersing ability moisture is not distributed to the skin. Yang moves quickly by nature and helps move this Qi around, so when astringency/dryness affect the body (especially the Lung), Yang cannot spread moisture and Wei Qi. Water may indeed be present in the body, but with no ability to disperse it, it sits without moving (edema). You might see Stomach gas, gurgling intestines, scanty watery menses, spotting and clotting during menstruation, weight retention, irritability, difficulty retaining a deep breath.
Dryness evil tends to attack the Lung	Five Element associated Lung with metal and dry. You can see this in the s/sx list too.

Signs and Symptoms of a Dryness Invasion

There are quite a few, but the first set is kind of a duh – all the s/sx are just various forms of dry. The second set is dryness + inability to send around the moisture that is there due to the astringent nature of dryness.

S/Sx of Dryness Invasion	Brief discussion
A bunch of dryness: • Dry skin • Dry eyes • Dry hair • Dry nose • Dry lips • Scanty urine • Dry cough with just a little bit of sticky	We discussed the heck out of this already. Scanty urine because of the lack of Body Fluids (dehydration). Skin might even be rough feeling and scaly.

mucus	
S/Sx of Dryness + Astringency affecting the Lung's moisture and Qi distribution functions	
• Stomach gas • Borborygmus • Scanty, watery menstruation • Spotting and small clots in menstrual bloods • Weight retention • Irritability • Difficulty retaining a breath	As stated before, this is beause there is actually plenty of moisture in the body, but the Lung Qi is affected by the astringent nature of the dryness, so it can no longer distribute the fluids properly.

Heat and Fire Evil

Heat and fire evils come from all seasons…except the summer heat season. There is a difference between heat and fire, but they are bundled together as they are both Yang and are sort of versions of the same thing. The difference between heat and fire is three-fold:

- Level of intensity
  Heat is the first stage. Fire is an advanced form of heat. Heat can develop *into* fire.

- Heat has general s/sx, Fire has more specific s/x
  o Heat.
    Think about the four bigs – big fever, great thirst, lots of sweating, and a forceful pulse. That is heat affecting the whole body.

  o Fire.
    This is a more specific and intense form of heat. Kind of like a fire ant bite – intense, localized, gets really red, develops a yellow pus, but doesn't generally affect the whole body. But it's definitely fire!

- Heat evil attacks the Qi while Fire attacks the Blood.

- Fire causes manic behavior due to it's affect upon the Heart and Blood. In the clinic, pus is always fire which is also called toxic heat.
- Heat attacks the Lung while Fire attacks the Pericardium, Heart, and Blood

Common Pathogenic Characteristics and Signs and Symptoms

Pay attention to this section and to the signs and symptoms therein.

Characteristics	Symptoms and Signs to know
Heat and fire are Yang pathogens and cause Yang Excess.	• Red face • High fever • Profuse sweating • Great thirst • Desire for cold drinks • Scanty, dark yellow urine that may burn upon release • Tongue = red body with a yellow coating • Pulse = fast, forceful, slippery Look at the four greats above: big fever, sweating, thirst and pulse. If this looks like the Summer Heat s/sx list, it is. But this can hit at any time of the year other than between Summer Solstice and Autumnal Equinox.
Heat and Fire evils consume Qi and Body Fluids causing Qi and Body Fluid deficiencies (again, this is like summer heat)	• All of the s/sx above, plus: • Fatigue and exhaustion fever burns off the body fluids/qi • Scanty urine and dry stool • Shortness of breath • Soft, weak voice
Heat and fire evils cause inner wind and bleeding	• Nasal bleeding • Bruising • Purpura • Bleeding gums • Etc…

	This is different than summer heat. Bleeding because heat, fire, and Yang pathogens make the blood flow faster and increase blood pressure. As you may know from biomedicine, the smaller capillaries in the body are a single layer of epithelial cells only held together by cellular junctions. Higher pressures can easily break those junctions causing blood leakage. Upper body bleeding is generally an excess while lower body bleeding is a deficiency.
Heat and fire can cause carbuncles and other skin problems	A carbuncle is a tight cluster of boils or a severe abscess and is generally infected with the staphylococcus bacteria. Generally red and raised with a palpable heat to it and the patient can often feel the pulse in this area. Skin cancer is also considered a form of toxic heat.

CHAPTER 14
Pathogenic Influences: Endogenous Pathogens

Endogenous is a pathology that results from conditions within the body rather than from an external influence. The previous chapter was about *exogenous* or exterior pathogens entering the body.

Endogenous pathogens in Chinese medicine refer to the five inner evils, Phlegm and Body Fluid retention, and Blood stagnation and Blood stasis.

THE FIVE INNER EVILS

Ok, really, the five both are and aren't evils: they aren't because they exist naturally in the body; they *are* when they become excessive due to the dysfunction of the internal organs. These evils are actually patterns and syndromes more than they are evils, but they manifest so similarly to the exterior invasions that they share names.

The five inner evils have the same pathological characteristics as the external evils of the same designation. They occur because of a dysfunction of the internal organs and can also flare as the result of toxic and chronic emotions.

Inner Evil	Brief discussion
Dampness	Look back at the symptoms of external damp evil discussion in the previous chapter. All of these apply to inner dampness as well. Look at the Spleen as one example of inner dampness, though other organs can be affected. Spleen functions best with conditions of moisture. When there is dysfunction of the Spleen, builds up dampness in the Middle Jiao causing all of the symptoms discussed in the previous chapter.

| Dry | See the section on external dryness. All of that applies here.

Lungs, Stomach, and Large Intestine are negatively impacted by dryness in the body. |
|-----|--|
| Cold | Inner cold is a more deficient cold, like a Yang deficiency. Exterior cold is an excess – an invasion of external cold.

Spleen and Kidney with a Yang deficiency will suffer inner cold. Yin pathogens cause Yang deficiencies leading to coagulation and contraction. |
| Heat | See the section on exterior heat invasions. All s/sx apply here.

Liver, Stomach and Heart are all susceptible to heat and fire. Heat can arise from stagnation and heat causes the next evil… |
| Wind | Wind in the body, like wind in the environment, occurs as the *result of heat* that is generated in some manner in the body.

Here's one example as to how that could occur: cold in the body causes contraction, which then leads to stagnation and stasis. This stagnant and static stuff leads to heat which leads to wind.

There are many fun ways this can occur. Blood deficiency is another way. Insufficient Blood volume leads to an insufficient blood flow which = stagnation then stasis, leading to heat, which leads to wind. |

Inner Wind is such a problem we need to discuss it further.

INNER WIND

Inner wind is not a pathogen, but a series of patterns we will talk about below. Treatment for each type is different, but all of them are considered nerve disorders. *All* inner wind is related to Liver and due to Liver. Why? Because Liver is the element of Wood and this is the element susceptible to wind. It just all just goes together.

Like wind in the environment, wind moves and changes quickly. Just last night I was sitting in my kitchen, typing away on this document. The air was totally still and hot one minute, then blowing so hard it was banging my kitchen windows open and shut the next. I had to scramble to shut them! Wind in the body can act like that too: arising out of seemingly nowhere very quickly, moving from place to place. As you study this section, look at how similar wind acts in the environment compared to how it acts in the body.

Inner wind is characterized by deviation of the mouth and tongue, seizures, tetany/shaking, convulsions, tremors of the extremities, twitching of the skin and more. This is caused by a dysfunction of the ligaments, tendons and sinews.

Liver controls these tissues, so inner wind is also called Liver Wind. The Liver also controls the nervous system including both the Peripheral Nervous System (PNS) and Central Nervous System (CNS). Dysfunction in these tissues manifests as seizures, numbness, and strokes. Liver controls the endocrine system as well. If a patient has excessive hormones, treat the Liver; if deficient hormones, treat the Kidney.

There are five causes of inner wind you need to know: extreme heat, Liver Yang rising, Liver or Kidney Yin deficiency, Blood deficiency, and Blood stasis. We will discuss each in detail below.

Inner wind caused by extreme heat

Things like acute tonsillitis, strep throat, and other problems caused by toxic heat (which is heat + pus) can generate inner wind.

All of these symptoms can also be caused by true heat with false cold. In biomedical-speak, this is shock due to infection. True heat with false cold has heat symptoms, but with low blood pressure, cold hands and feet. Still need to treat the heat and when that is corrected will also fix the false cold.

I'll give you a symptom list to know….but it's unlikely you'll see all of these at once! If you do, you've stumbled into a remake of the Exorcist! Run!

S/sx of Inner Wind due to Extreme Heat	Brief discussion
Onset: acute	Quick moving nature of wind
Pt has a history of catching cold	Compromised immunity, exterior heat/Yang invasion
Sore throat due to excessive Yang s/sx	
Convulsions	Wind influence
Upward staring eyes	
Semi-consciousness	
Tetany	
Stiff neck and extremities	
Stiff tongue	
Manic behavior	Heat s/sx
Restlessness	
Delirium	
Pulse: wiry	Reflection of the Liver involvement
Tongue: red body with yellow coating	Heat s/sx

Inner wind caused by Liver Yang rising

This is a "wind stroke" in Chinese medicine – a cerebrovascular attack caused by hypertension.

Note that a history of hypertension and dizziness, vertigo, and a throbbing headache. These are early warning signs. Blood pressure of 150/90 is the *top range of functionality*—anything above these numbers is really critical and is called toxic high blood pressure or toxic hypertension. Always take your patients' blood pressure. If it is over these numbers, *refer them to an MD* and note it on the patient history. They might have accompanying signs of double vision, and dizziness.

S/sx of Inner Wind due to Lv Yang rising	Brief discussion
History of hypertension and dizziness, vertigo, and a throbbing headache	These are the precursor conditions – the early warning signs.
Suddenly falls down	Not constantly, just conscious and upright one minute, falling down and unconscious the next.
Loss of consciousness	
Deviation of mouth and tongue	All are signs and symptoms of stroke in western medicine. Aphasia is in ability to speak or speak correctly. Hemiplegia is paralysis or weakness affecting one side of the body.
One side of the nasolabial groove disappears	
Tongue is stiff and trembles	
Aphasia	
Hemplegia	

Inner wind caused by Liver and/or Kidney Yin deficiency

This is a long term problem generated by the chronic condition of Yin deficiency of the Liver and/or Kidney. Liver and Kidney are BFFs, besties, friends for life, so when one suffers the other generally does too. All of the signs and symptoms below can be accompanied by Yin deficieny s/sx such as ear ringing, deafness, lower back pain, a tongue that is thin and may have cracking and trembles, and a thin wiry pulse.

When you read through the s/sx list below, this should remind you of Parkinson's Disease.

S/sx of Inner Wind due to Lv and/or Ki Yin deficiency	Brief discussion
Joint stiffness	Liver and Kidneys feed the sinews and tendons. Unable to do this, the body experiences the stiffness, tightness, and tetany.
Neck stiffness	
Natural cervical spine curve straightens	
"Mask face"	No facial expressions or eye blinks because of the stiffness in the muscles and tendons.
Eyes do not blink	
Resting tremors	The body trembles when the patient is still – wind influence

Staggering gait Turns around in tiny steps	Takes tiny steps because of the stiffness and tetany
Handwriting progresss from large to tiny when writing a sentence	Tendons and muscles in the arm and hand get stiffer and stiffer with use.
Pill rolling hand motions	Characteristic Parkinson's sign. Patient will make a motion like rolling a pill between their thumb and forefinger at a rate of about 3 times per second.

Inner wind caused by Blood deficiency

One example of Blood deficiency is anemia. Women with heavy bleeding during their periods might also experience the s/sx below. The wind generated by Blood deficiency is clearly not as severe as the s/sx above.

S/sx of Inner Wind due to Blood Deficiency	Brief discussion
History of Blood xu	Look for all of the Blood xu s/sx: pale nails, pale face and lips, scanty menstruation, etc.
Numbness of extremities	Fingers and toes, specifically. This follows the history of Blood deficiency.
Skin twitching	Or even the sensation of twitching. This is also called "worm walking" – the sensation of a small insect walking on the skin.
Spasms of the extremities	Especially during the night and especially the calves.
Floaters in the vision	Spots you see when you look at a clear blue sky, a white wall. They seem to float around in the vision field.
Dizziness and vertigo	Especially dizziness upon standing
Tongue: small, pale, thin coating Pulse: thin and weak	Common presentations in Blood xu.

Inner wind caused by Blood stasis

Will you find this in your Maciocia book? Nope. This comes courtesy of Dr. Qianzhi Wu, my Foundations professor. This generally results after an accident, especially head trauma, with subjective concussion symptoms such as nausea, dizziness, memory loss, vertigo, all wind symptoms. An objective symptom would be resulting secondary epilepsy due to the accident. (Primary epilepsy is from childhood, not due to a traceable cause.)

The s/sx below are the same as Qi Closing or Qi Tense Syndrome. If the loss of consciousness lasts more than 5 minutes, call 911. (If the patient is not breathing, obviously call a whole lot faster.)

Inner Wind s/sx due to Blood stasis	Brief discussion
Upward staring eyes	See the Qi Closing or Qi Tense Syndrome write up in Chapter 2.
Clenched jaws	
Clenched lips	
Screaming like a sheep or pig	I still have no frame of reference for this....
Pulse: wiry	
Tongue: stiff	

PHLEGM AND BODY FLUID RETENTION

Phlegm and Body Fluid retention are disorders of body fluid metabolism caused by dysfunction of the Spleen, Kidney, and Lung (the three organs responsible for body fluid metabolism). The Spleen is the most important of these three. When the Spleen is out of balance it loses its ability to fully control the transportation of food and water in the body. A kind of swampiness results as the water of the body stagnates, resulting in inner dampness.

Phlegm is produced by either pathological heat or pathological cold plus dampness. Pathological heat will "cook" the damp down into the sticky phlegm. While pathological cold will congeal the damp into a kind of internal slushee that produces phlegm, the more likely scenario with dampness + cold is that it becomes Body Fluid retention.

Dampness + ...	Discussion
Pathological heat = phlegm	Pathological heat from Lung or Stomach when combined with damp = phlegm. Frequently eating greasy, fried foods, for instance, can create pathological Stomach fire which heats the damp and leads to phlegm. Smoking (cigarettes, cigars, pot, whatever) will introduce toxic heat into the Lung, cooking the damp and making phlegm. Lung disharmony is the most likely cause for pathological heat leading to phlegm.
Pathological cold = Body Fluid retention	Usually.....later on you will talk about cold phlegm and hot phlegm in your herb classes. But in this case, know that damp + cold usually results in Body Fluid retention. If damp is cooled by a Spleen Yang deficiency or a Kidney Yang deficiency, you'll likely see water retention or edema (aka Body Fluid retention) in the lower body. Kidney disharmony is most likely of the two possibilities above.

Phlegm Retention

Phlegm is sticky – stickier than damp – and likely to hang on in the body. While phlegm in the western medical system is a measurable quantity of good, phlegm in the Chinese medical model can be both *visible* (like you see in biomedicine) and *invisible*. Let's compare the two.

Type of phlegm	Brief discussion
Visible phlegm	This is phlegm in the *Lung*. Symptoms are a tight feeling in the chest and coughing up mucus in the morning. Stroke patients often have a lot of mucus with hoarse breathing. Dirty, sticky phlegm in the Lung.
Invisible phlegm	You can't see this or measure it, but you can see the results of phlegm in the channels and in the brain. • In the channels: Nodules in the neck and throat, swollen lymph nodes. All of these will be soft and may or may not have pain. • In the brain: Foggy thinking or unclear thinking, poor memory, confusion. Many mental health problems in China are attributed to invisible phlegm.

Signs and Symptoms of Phlegm Retention

Signs and symptoms change depending on whether the organs or channels are affected. The most likely organs to be affected by phlegm retention are the Lung, Stomach (or Middle Jiao), and Heart. Know the signs and symptoms!

Phlegm in the Lung

S/sx of Phlegm in the Lung	Brief discussion
Cough with profuse white or yellow mucus	White when affected by cold, yellow when coupled with heat
Chest tightness or distention	Caused by the sticky phlegm impacting the breath
Asthma	Wheezing and all noisy breathing related symptoms are a result of rebellious Lung qi passing through phlegm.
Wheezing	
Dyspnea	Difficulty breathing. You can have this with or without asthma.
Shortness of breath	Also abbreviated SOB.
Tongue: swollen body with teethmarks, coating is greasy/dirty and either white or yellow	Swollen indicates Body Fluid retention. Teethmarks are the result of edema on the tongue. Coating will be yellow when heat is present.
Pulse: slippery and/or wiry	

Phlegm in the Middle Jiao

Any s/sx you see above the umbilicus are upper digestive disorders – Stomach. If you see s/sx below the umbilicus, those are lower digestive disorders – Spleen.

S/sx of Phlegm in the Middle Jiao	Brief discussion
Nausea	Phlegm causing an inability of the Stomach to descend Qi.
Vomiting	
Retching	
Belching	
Fullness in the Stomach	Due to the presence of phlegm in the Middle Jiao.
Low appetite	
Tongue: swollen body with teethmarks, coating is greasy/dirty and either white or yellow	Swollen indicates Body Fluid retention. Teeth marks are the result of edema on the tongue and the tongue pressing against the teeth. Coating will be yellow when heat is present.
Pulse: slippery and/or wiry	

Phlegm in the Heart

OK, really it's phlegm affecting the Heart. Notice the heart + damp signs in this list.

S/sx of Phlegm in the Heart	Brief discussion
Tossing and turning at night Poor sleep or insomnia	Heart related stuff. Restlessness, in other words. Poor sleep and insomnia is kind of an exacerbation of sleep problems
Forgetfulness or poor memory	Also a heart related symptom, but damp/phlegm can make this worse.
Confusion Heavy headedness Sleepiness Foggy mind	Damp signs. Sleepiness here indicates that this patient wants 10-12 hours of sleep. Maybe more.
Tongue: swollen body with teethmarks, coating is greasy/dirty and either white or yellow Pulse: slippery and/or wiry	Swollen indicates Body Fluid retention. Teeth marks are the result of edema on the tongue and the tongue pressing against the teeth. Coating will be yellow when heat is present.

Phlegm in the Channels

S/sx of Phlegm in the Channels	Brief discussion
Swelling in the extremities Lymphomas Nodules Swollen lymph nodes	Localized, no known reason, not edema. Lymphomas, nodules, swollen lymph nodes are all types of swelling in the extremities.
Tongue: swollen body with teethmarks, coating is greasy/dirty and either white or yellow Pulse: slippery and/or wiry	Swollen indicates Body Fluid retention. Teeth marks are the result of edema on the tongue and the tongue pressing against the teeth. Coating will be yellow when heat is present.

Body Fluid Retention

In *The Golden Chamber* Zhang Zhongjing says there are four types of Body Fluid retention. Remember that thing about the word <u>Yin meaning Body Fluid</u> in Chinese? You'll see that reflected in the names of the four types below.

Four types of BFluid retention	Brief discussion
Taiyin	Water retention in the Lung. As the upper source of water, when Lung cannot descend or disperse, you see this: • Edema in the face and eyelids and upper extremities • Puffy eyes • Coughing up loose watery mucus • Drainage and post nasal drip • Pulmonary edema
Yuanyin	Water retention in the chest wall/hypochondria This shows in an X-ray. In biomed they use a needle to remove the fluid retention then they put meds in to assist with fluid resolution. S/sx look like this: • Coughing with chest pain • Hard to lie flat due to the pain • Pain increases when body twists • Shortness of breath (SOB)
Yiyin	Retention of water under the skin – generalized edema Can happen anywhere on the body, but most likely to happen on the lower extremities, especially around the ankles and dorsum of the foot. Press on the skin with your thumb for a few seconds to test for "pitting edema". If the skin does not return back to its normal state within about 60 seconds, it's probably water edema. There is also a kind of edema called Qi edema. Swelling, but not pitting.

Zhiyin	Water retention in the Stomach
	Nausea, vomiting, and morning sickness are all possible here. The vomit will be watery and loose and is likely to be accompanied by hiccups, epigastric fullness, and loud noises in the intestines. Water retention here is suppressing the Stomach's natural descending abilities.

BLOOD STAGNATION AND BLOOD STASIS

Blood stagnation (or Xue Yu) is the process of Blood flowing more slowly in the body than it is supposed to flow. This is a process as much as it is a condition/syndrome. Left unchecked, it leads to Blood stasis.

Blood stasis (aka Yu Xue) is when Blood *stops* flowing altogether. Blood stasis is a visible phenomenon, visible on CT scans, Xrays, and MRIs. Blood stasis is also a syndrome description with definable signs and symptoms.

It's important to understand that there is a clear difference between Blood stagnation and Blood stasis. Stagnation is a condition and an ongoing issue that *develops* into Blood stasis. Stasis is an endogenous: it causes new problems and is the *result* of stagnation. Of the two, Blood Stasis is the more serious condition with the poorer prognosis.

Etiologies of Blood Stagnation and Blood Stasis

There are three causes to know. Always pay attention to what *causes* the condition of Blood stagnation or Blood stasis. You have to know what caused it in order to effectively treat it.

Three etiologies	Brief discussion
Cold in the Blood	This cold can originate externally or internally. Cold contracts the tissues and Blood channels, causing coagulation. This is also why the skin become pale and then blue when it gets cold.

Heat in the Blood	Four reasons this affect Blood this way:
	• Heat in the Blood can raise blood pressure to the point that the Blood leaks out of the capillaries and vessels.
	• Can dry Body Fluids making the Blood thicker and thicker.
	• Heat can consume Qi, causing Qi deficiency.
	• Pathogens fight against the Upright Qi inside the vessels, which can also block Blood flow. Old Chinese medical literature refers to the pathogens as "ghosts" so you will sometimes see this reference when you read about the fight between Upright Qi and pathogenic influences.
Qi disorders	Qi is the force that moves Blood. A Qi deficiency will cause the Blood to move more slowly. A Qi stagnation (like Liver Qi stagnation) will cause Blood stagnation for the same reason. And then, of course, once the Blood is slowed and stagnant, it can easily progress to Blood stasis.

Signs and Symptoms of Blood Stagnation and Blood Stasis

Please be clear: these are symptoms and signs of a Blood stagnation/stasis problem, not a Qi stagnation problem.

S/Sx of Blood Stasis/Stagnation	Brief discussion
Pain • Fixed, not moving • Worse at night • Worse when it's cold • Sharp	Note the *nature* of the pain. Different types of stagnation have different qualities of pain. (*Qi* stagnation, for instance is distending pain and wanders.) The sharpness of the pain is often described as stabbing or pins and needles.

Bleeding • Dark in color • Bleeding out of vessels	Color is generally dark red, purple, brownish. Menstrual bleeding colors will be similar and there will likely be either large or small clots. Bleeding out of the vessels can be something somewhat milder like purpura and bruising or something more severe like cerebral bleeding, embolism, thrombosis.
Masses or bruises	Bruising would be caused by trauma of some kind. Masses are more internal and not due to trauma. This includes cancerous masses.
Tongue s/sx • Purple tongue body • Purple spots on tongue	In Chapter 3 we talked a lot about blood stagnation and stasis and mentioned this tongue presentation in detail. Please review that.
Pulse s/sx	Again, I refer you to Chapter 3.

This page intentionally left blank

CHAPTER 15
Mechanisms of Disease, Diagnostics, and Treatment Strategies

MECHANISMS OF DISEASE

Disease is a process of fighting between pathogens and upright (Zheng) Qi, resulting in disharmony or imbalance of the body. Disease can be functional or organic.

- Functional disease only affects the channels and Qi/energy flow. Functional diseases show negative results in laboratory tests.
- Organic causes affect the Blood and internal organs. Organic diseases show in tests as viruses, bacterial infections, etc. Organic diseases develop from functional problems.

Excess and deficiency syndromes

There are two terms that define the *percentage* of Zheng/Upright Qi and the *percentage* of pathogen: excess and deficiency. It's sort of the Chinese medicine version of a football score to determine who is currently ahead in the game.

Excess syndromes

In an excess syndrome, the Zheng Qi and the pathogen are both strong, resulting in severe symptoms and a strong reaction. Symptoms might include stuff like the four bigs, a cough with yellow mucus, etc.

Deficiency syndromes

In a deficiency syndrome, the Zheng Qi is weak and wimp. The pathogen could be either strong or weak. Either way, with a weak Upright/Zheng Qi, the fight will be minimal, so the reaction will be mild.

This is kind of like having a very bad football team – they lose so easily that there is very little drama when they do so.

Treatment is to to tonify the deficiency of the Zheng Qi. Will this also tonify the pathogen? Most likely, but if the Zheng Qi gets stronger this is still ok. Note that this will intensify the fight and thus the symptoms because both fighters are now stronger. Once the Zheng Qi is strong you can then sedate the pathogen. The Zheng Qi may even do this on it's own.

Gauging Excess and Deficiency Syndromes

The disease processes as described here applies to all diseases. You put percentages on how much excess or deficiency there is to help determine your treatment plan – will you tonify the deficiency or sedate the excess? These measurements also help determine how big the fight between the Zheng Qi and the pathogen is.

Excess

An excess is generally the acute phase of disease. This is where the pathogen invades and the s/sx start.

Combination of Excess and Deficiency

The middle stage of a disease. There are three possible scenarios here:
- More excess, less deficiency
- More deficiency, less excess
- Half deficiency, half excess

Deficiency

This is the late or chronic stage of disease. If it lasts this long, deficiency is now running the show.

Yin and Yang Disorders

We covered these in some depth in the first book, (*Chinese Medicine 101: Start with the Foundations*, available on Amazon in both digital and print formats.). I would refer you to that for a full discussion on Yin and Yang disorders.

Yin and Yang can suffer excesses or deficiencies. Excesses generally characterize the acute stage of a disease while deficiencies are the chronic stage of a disease. "Acute" is defined in various ways, but as a general rule, anything a patient has had for 21 days or less is acute. If the condition lasts longer than that it is then in the chronic stage.

What follows is a brief review of Yin and Yang signs and symptoms of excesses and deficiencies.

Yang Excess S/Sx	Yin Excess S/Sx
• The four greats (thirst, sweat, pulse, fever) • Speaking loudly • Manic behavior • Forceful pulse • Red tongue body with yellow coating	• History of common cold • Chills with aversion to cold • Cold pain • Warming therapies have no affect on the cold s/sx • No sweating • Superficial, tight pulse • Normal tongue
Yang Deficiency S/Sx	Yin Deficiency S/Sx
• Pale face • Cold extremities • Cold can be alleviated with warming therapies • Watery diarrhea • Cold pain with a desire for warming • Tongue is pale, swollen body, moist wet coating • Pulse is deep, weak, slow.	• Night sweats • Palm Heat (hot sensation in palms and soles of feet) • Tidal fever (late afternoon fever) • Red on the face only in the zygomatic area, rest of face is pale. • Hot flashes • Tongue body is red, thin, probably has cracks. Little to no tongue coating

To diagnose a condition as either a Yin or Yang disease you have to determine if there's hot or cold and if the condition is excess or deficient. Example: hyperthyroid is a Yin deficiency and generates a lot of heat. Hypothyroid is a Yang deficiency of either Spleen or Kidney and generates an awful lot of cold.

You'll get lots more about this in further Diagnosis studies.

DIAGNOSTICS BASICS

There are many diagnostics models available to you in Chinese medicine. You'll cover them more thoroughly in the diagnostics full modules later on.

The model for diagnosing we will talk about here is the Eight Principles method. It's quick, down and dirty, and is the simplest one I know. For this you think in pairs: exterior/interior, hot/cold, excess/deficiency, and finally Yin/Yang. You go through these pairs one at a time, add up what you've got, and make a determination.

When you are super stuck in clinic and don't know *what* is going on, default to this to get you pointed in the right direction. Ask these questions about the patient after you've done your intake and interview and do it in this order:

1.	What is the location of the problem in the body?	a. Exterior b. Interior
2.	What kind of temperature presentations am I seeing?	a. Heat b. Cold
3.	Is the current situation showing excess or deficiency s/sx?	a. Excess b. Deficiency

If you look back at your answers and find you answered all A's, you are looking at an Exterior Heat Excess – aka, a Yang Excess. If it's all B's it's an Interior Cold Deficiency. What if the answers are mixed?

So this is just one little brief glimpse into diagnosis. To get a really complete treatment diagnosis, you need seven components:
1. A western medical diagnosis
2. Chinese disease name
3. Differential diagnosis, pattern differentiation, or syndrome

4. Location of disease
5. Property of disease (external/internal, heat/cold, excess/deficiency)
6. Principles of treatment
7. Acupuncture point prescription, herbal formulas, other treatments

TCM TREATMENT PRINCIPLES

Four treatment principles will get you a very basic understanding of the information you will expand on at length later on.

Tonify Upright/Zheng Qi and body constitution while sedating pathogens

Disease is a process of fighting between Zheng Qi and pathogens. You have to know when to sedate, when to tonify.

Problem	What to do
Single excess?	Sedate it.
Single deficiency?	Tonify it.
Combination of excess and deficiency?	Now that's far more likely! Treatment depends on the situation • More excess, less deficiency o Sedate first, then tonify • More deficiency, less excess o Tonify first, then sedate • Half deficiency, half excess o Tonify and sedate simultaneously

Using cancer as an example, in the US, the survival rate is lower than in China or Japan. In these countries a DOM (doc of oriental med) is involved in treatment in addition to Western cancer therapies. The DOM gets the patient stronger with herbs and acupuncture prior to chemo and radation treatment as afterwards so that the body takes a smaller hit from the toxins involved in treatment which lower the body's strength. As an acupuncturist you can make a plan for the patient. Radiation and chemotherapy is a sedation type therapy. On OM doc follows up with Shi Guan Da Bu Tang is a tonifying treatment to help the body recover. The combination of treatment types improves the quality of a person's life and increases survival rates.

Regulate Yin and Yang

How to regulate Yin/Yang	Brief version of how
Sedate Yang excesses	Through blood letting, gua sha, wet cupping, cold herbs
Sedate Yin excesses	Moxibustion in the upper body, acrid and pungent herbs
Tonify Yin deficiencies	Use herbs, acupoints on the lower Yin channels (Sp, Lv, Ki). You can use dietary therapies to build the Blood and Essence and Yin (like salmon, for instance).
Tonify Yang deficiencies	Use warm herbs and dietary therapy (shrimp, coffee, and other Yang tonification foods.

Distinguish the root from the branch

The root or the *ben* in Chinese medicine is the cause of the disease. The symptoms and signs are referred to as *biao*.

- In an emergency or acute situation, treat the *biao*, the symptoms and signs.
  Using acute asthma as an example, treat the signs and symptoms causing distress: shortness of breath and wheezing.

- In chronic situations, you treat the *ben* or the root of the problem.
  Using asthma again, treat the root when the patient is in between acute attacks.

Treat disease according to climatic and geographic conditions as well as individual constitution

In Spring for instance, focus on removing wind from the upper body. Depression is worse in Yin seasons of fall and winter. For men, work on the Kidneys and for women work on the Liver. Gender, age, etc. all affect treatment.

Tailor make herbs whenever possible for individual constitutions. As a rule, that's better than pre-fab patent formulas.

This page intentionally left blank

ABOUT THE AUTHOR

Cat Calhoun is a licensed acupuncture practitioner in the State of Texas and soon to be in the State of Florida as well. She attended AOMA Graduate School of Integrative Medicine, earning a Masters degree in Acupuncture and Oriental Medicine. She is passionate about teaching, both formally and informally. Cat has single-handedly created and managed CatsTCMNotes.com since 2008, dispensing notes and clinical pearls to students and practitioners for the past 11 years. She is also passionate about learning, and is currently in love with Master Tung's Acupuncture system.

This book, *Chinese Medicine 101: Start with the foundations*, has a companion book for the 2nd half of your Foundational education in Chinese medicine. Look for it Amazon: *Chinese Medicine 102: Complete your foundations*. Both of these books are vital for framing your understanding of the philosophy and basic understanding of Chinese medicine.